General Practice Nursing
Foundational principles

For the full range of M&K Publishing books please visit our website:
ww.mkupdate.co.uk

General Practice Nursing
Foundational principles

Edited by Deborah Duncan

General Practice Nursing: Foundational principles
Deborah Duncan

ISBN: 978-1-910451-21-2

First published 2019

Reprinted 2021

All rights reserved. No part of this publication may be reproduced, stored in a retrieval system, or transmitted in any form or by any means, electronic, mechanical, photocopying, recording or otherwise, without either the prior permission of the publishers or a licence permitting restricted copying in the United Kingdom issued by the Copyright Licensing Agency, 90 Tottenham Court Road, London, W1T 4LP. Permissions may be sought directly from M&K Publishing, phone: 01768 773030, fax: 01768 781099 or email: publishing@mkupdate.co.uk

Any person who does any unauthorised act in relation to this publication may be liable to criminal prosecution and civil claims for damages.

British Library Cataloguing in Publication Data

A catalogue record for this book is available from the British Library

Notice

Clinical practice and medical knowledge constantly evolve. Standard safety precautions must be followed, but, as knowledge is broadened by research, changes in practice, treatment and drug therapy may become necessary or appropriate. Readers must check the most current product information provided by the manufacturer of each drug to be administered and verify the dosages and correct administration, as well as contraindications. It is the responsibility of the practitioner, utilising the experience and knowledge of the patient, to determine dosages and the best treatment for each individual patient. Any brands mentioned in this book are as examples only and are not endorsed by the publisher. Neither the publisher nor the authors assume any liability for any injury and/or damage to persons or property arising from this publication.

To contact M&K Publishing write to:
M&K Update Ltd · The Old Bakery · St. John's Street
Keswick · Cumbria CA12 5AS
Tel: 01768 773030 · Fax: 01768 781099
publishing@mkupdate.co.uk
www.mkupdate.co.uk

Designed and typeset by Mary Blood
Printed by Bell & Bain, Glasgow

Contents

List of figures vii
List of tables vii
List of boxes vii
Acknowledgements x
List of abbreviations xi
Introduction xiii

1 The role of the GPN: Political, professional and economic drivers 1
  Deborah Duncan

2 Consultation skills 11
  Deborah Duncan

3 Public health and an introduction to health screening 17
  Deborah Duncan

4 Cervical cytology 27
  Sian Hayes and Deborah Duncan

5 Women's health 35
  Deborah Duncan

6 Men's health 45
  Deborah Duncan

7 Immunisation 55
  Jacqueline Johnstone

8 Travel health 69
  Deborah Duncan

9 Ear care 77
  Sian Hayes and Deborah Duncan

10 Wound care 85
  Nuala McCarron

11 General principles of long-term conditions 97
  Deborah Duncan

12 Diabetes 107
  Sian Hayes

13 **Respiratory conditions** 133
   Deborah Duncan

14 **Chronic kidney disease** 151
   Evelyn Walton

15 **Coronary heart disease** 157
   Evelyn Walton

16 **Cancer as a long-term condition** 173
   Deborah Duncan

17 **Dementia** 181
   Deborah Duncan

18 **Mental illness as a long-term condition** 189
   Deborah Duncan

19 **Conclusion** 197
   Deborah Duncan

   Index 203

List of figures

Figure 4.1: Taking a smear 33
Figure 6.1: Goserelin acetate (Zoladex) being administered 48
Figure 6.2: Self-examination of the testes 51
Figure 7.1: Department of Health 'Vaccination Planner' 63
Figure 10.1: Layers of the skin 87
Figure 11.1: House of Care model 102
Figure 12.1: Healthier you 112
Figure 15.1: Management of hypertension 160

List of tables

Table 6.1: Risk stratification for men with localised prostate cancer 47
Table 7.1: NHS childhood vaccine coverage statistics 57
Table 7.2: Childhood MMR vaccine coverage 57
Table 7.3: Diseases that we immunise against 60
Table 7.4: Immunisation schedule for infants aged up to 1 year 64
Table 7.5: Selective immunisation schedule for infants 65
Table 7.6: Management of potential side effects 66
Table 9.1: Methods of ear wax removal 80
Table 10.1: Factors that affect wound healing 88
Table 10.2: Exudate 91
Table 10.3: Dressing selection 92
Table 12.1: WHO recommendations diagnostic criteria for diabetes 108
Table 12.2: Diagnosing type 2 diabetes 110
Table 13.1: The MRC dyspnoea scale 140
Table 13.2: Clinical features of asthma and COPD 140
Table 14.1: Prognosis of CKD by GFR and albuminuria categories 153
Table 15.1: New York Heart Association (NYHA) functional classification of heart failure 165

List of boxes

Box 1.1: The Queen's Nursing Institute 5
Box 1.2: Reader activity – timeline 8
Box 1.3: Resources 8
Box 2.1: The NMC code and communication 12
Box 2.2: Reader activity – models of consultation 15

Box 3.1: The role of Public Health England 19
Box 3.2: The responsibilities of Public Health Wales 21
Box 3.3: Reader activity – policy documents 22
Box 3.4: Reader activity – health promotion theory 24
Box 3.5: Answers to reader activity – health promotion theory 25
Box 4.1: Reader activity – timeline 28
Box 4.2: Screening ages 29
Box 5.1: Reader activity – types of contraception 38
Box 5.2: Breast care 41
Box 5.3: Resources 42
Box 5.4: Answers to reader activity – types of contraception 42
Box 6.1: Reader activity – Goserelin acetate 48
Box 6.2: Self-examination of the testes 51
Box 6.3: Resources 52
Box 6.4: Erectile dysfunction pathway 53
Box 7.1: Reader activity – case study 58
Box 7.2: Reader activity – questions 60
Box 7.3: Resources 66
Box 8.1: Anti-malarials 74
Box 8.2: Resources 75
Box 9.1: Self-management ear care advice from NICE 79
Box 9.3: Reader activity – ear syringing 81
Box 9.4: Answers to reader activity – ear syringing 82
Box 9.5: Resources 82
Box 10.1: Reader activity – ulcers 89
Box 10.2: Reader activity – wound infection 93
Box 10.3: Resources 94
Box 10.4: Answers to reader activity – wound infection 94
Box 11.1: Aspects of self-care 98
Box 11.2 Reader activity – action plans 101
Box 11.3: Key points from Liberating the NHS 102
Box 11.4: Resources 103
Box 12.1: Reader activity – case study 1 108
Box 12.2: Reader activity – case study 2 110
Box 12.3: Reader activity – diabetes education 115
Box 12.4: Reader activity – bariatric surgery 115
Box 12.5: Patient factors 116

Box 12.6: NICE diabetes management recommendations 117
Box 12.7: Reader activity – further review 119
Box 12.8: Reader activity – Exercise referral 121
Box 12.9: Key recommendations 122
Box 12.10: Reader activity – further review 128
Box 12.11: Reader activity – differential diagnosis 129
Box 12.12: Answers to reader activity – further review 130
Box 13.1: Reader activity – flu vaccine 136
Box 13.2: Fractional exhaled nitric oxide 139
Box 13.3: Inhaler devices 146
Box 13.4: Answers to reader activity – flu vaccine 147
Box 13.5: Resources 148
Box 14.1: Resources 155
Box 15.1: Reader activity 164
Box 15.2: Resources 168
Box 16.1: The stepwise approach to pain relief 176
Box 16.2: Definitions of depression 177
Box 16.3: Resources 178
Box 17.1: Criteria used when diagnosing dementia subtypes 184
Box 17.2: The different types of dementia 184
Box 17.3: Additional tests for specific diagnosis 185
Box 17.4: Reader activity – dementia services 186
Box 17.5: Resources 187
Box 18.1: Reader activity – mental illness 191
Box 18.2: Different types of mental illness 192
Box 18.3: Resources 193
Box 19.1: Reader activity – patient group directions 200
Box 19.2: Resources 202

Acknowledgements

I want to thank my friends and colleagues at Bucks New University, particularly Abigail Ashby, Sue Axe and Agnes Fanning. A big thank you too for the staff at the School of Nursing and Midwifery at Queen's University Belfast; and to Katherine Rodgers for her ongoing support. I also want to thank all the individuals involved in writing this book: Sian Hayes, Jacqueline Johnstone, Evelyn Waugh and Nuala McCarron.

Then I also want to thank my friends and family, namely my husband Malcolm and Matthew, Benjamin, Anna, Riodhna, Eve, Elizabeth, Jacob, Rob and Emily. Thank you all for your patience while I was writing this book.

Deborah Duncan

List of abbreviations

A1AT alpha-1 antitrypsin
ACEi angiotensin-converting enzyme inhibitor
ACOS asthma-COPD overlap syndrome
ACR albumin to creatinine ratio
ACVD atherosclerotic cardiovascular disease
ARBs angiotensin11 receptor antagonists
AF atrial fibrillation

BDR bronchodilator reversibility
BMI body mass index
BP blood pressure

Ca cancer
CCG clinical commissioning group
CKD chronic kidney disease
COPD chronic obstructive pulmonary disease
CT computed tomography
CVD cardiovascular disease

DKA diabetic ketoacidosis

ECG electrocardiogram
eGFR estimated glomerular filtration rate
ESR erythrocyte sedimentation rate

FBC full blood count
FEF forced expiratory flow
FENO fractional exhaled nitric oxide
FEV forced expiratory volume
GP General Practitioner
GPN General Practice Nurse

HaH Hospital at Home
Hb haemoglobin.
HbA1c average blood glucose (sugar) level
HCA healthcare assistant
HEE Health Education England
HF heart failure
HHS hyperosmolar hyperglycaemic state
HPV human papilloma virus

IHSs inhaled steroids
INR international normalised ratio blood test
LABAs long-acting beta-agonists
LAMAs long-acting muscarinic receptor antagonists
LBC liquid-based cytology
LDL low-density lipoprotein
LFTs liver function tests
LLN lower limit of normal (in airflow limitation)
MI myocardial infarction
NHS National Health Service
NHSCSP NHS Cervical Screening Programme
NOACs non-vitamin K antagonist oral anticoagulants
NSAIDs nonsteroidal anti-inflammatory drugs
QNI Queen's Nursing Institute
QOF Qualities Outcome Framework
PGD patient group direction
PHE Public Health England
PSD patient specific direction
RCGP Royal College of General Practitioners
SABAs short-acting beta agonists
SAMAs short-acting muscarinic antagonists
SGLT2i sodium-glucose transport protein 2 inhibitors
SLE systemic lupus erythematosus
SUs sulphonylureas
T2D type 2 diabetes
U&Es urea and electrolytes
VC vital capacity
WHO World Health Organization

Introduction

The role of the General Practice Nurse (GPN) has changed rapidly over the past few decades. GPNs now play a key part in primary care, relieving General Practitioners of much of their previous workload (Baird *et al.* 2016). Predicted changes in the GPN workforce have also led to much interest in – and financial support for – this branch of nursing across the UK.

This book is written for nurses who want to work in primary care and for those who are new to the GPN role or returning to it after a long gap. The content aligns with the Queen's Nursing Institute (2015) and Health Education England (2017) competency framework. Across the different countries in the UK, the existing framework is being revisited to ensure that these competencies also match each local area's requirements. For instance, in Northern Ireland nurses are employed as treatment room staff as well as GPNs.

This book aims to support the student who is learning the foundational skills needed to develop into a confident and competent primary care nurse. It therefore provides relevant information about clinical skills and knowledge, health promotion and screening, and the management and assessment of long-term conditions. Some topics have been omitted or only mentioned in passing because the GPN will require additional training in order to tackle them properly. For instance, some aspects of women's sexual health are discussed in Chapters 4 and 5 but further reading will clearly be required to gain an in-depth knowledge of this complex subject.

Scattered through the text, you will see boxed reader's activities, which are designed to reinforce the content. These activities may require you to draw a timeline or make notes, for instance. You should therefore keep a notebook close at hand so that you can complete the activities and check your answers when they appear, later in the text.

References

Baird, B., Charles A., Honeyman, M., *et al.* (2016). *Understanding pressures in general practice.* London: King's Fund.

Health Education England (2017). *The General Practice Workforce Development Plan.*

Queen's Nursing Institute (QNI) (2015). *District Nursing and General Practice Nursing Service Education and Career Framework.* https://www.hee.nhs.uk/sites/default/files/documents/Interactive%20version%20of%20the%20framework_1.pdf (last accessed 5.2.2019).

Chapter 1

The role of the GPN: Political, professional and economic drivers

Deborah Duncan

Introduction

In all corners of the NHS, work is currently being undertaken to develop a robust competency framework for both treatment room nurses and general practice nurses. This chapter looks at how the GPN role has changed since the 1960s.

Historically, GPNs contributed to the delivery of the GP contract to the whole spectrum of the practice population. Now GPNs work as part of a multi-disciplinary team (MDT) within GP surgeries, assessing, screening and treating patients of all ages. They also offer health promotion advice in areas such as contraception, weight loss, smoking cessation and travel health. Their role now also embraces expertise in long-term conditions (LTCs), preventative services, sexual health and advanced clinical skills (QNI 2015). There is a specific skill set to manage uncertainty and risk when supporting people who may have undifferentiated diagnoses. All this has to be delivered according to guidelines and protocols, adhering to the Quality Outcomes Framework (QOF) within general practice. Nurses will be central to the delivery of the new care model set out in the *NHS' Five Years Forward View* (NHS 2014) so that they can meet the needs of an ageing population, many of whom have comorbidities and long-term conditions (Goodwin et al. 2011).

In 1948, when the NHS was created, GPNs were responsible for all personal medical care. They became the gateway for individuals to access hospitals, specialist care and social care. In the early days of the NHS there were few explicit standards for general practice, and few incentives for medical professionals to take on the GP role (Godwin et al. 2011). There was also a rapidly growing demand for services (Collings 1950). Many GP practices employed nurses to support them with these challenges.

The 1960s to the 1980s

The role of the GPN then saw significant financial support and development in the 1960s. The first contract between General Practitioners (GPs) and the NHS was formalised in 1966 and this covered funding for ancillary staff, including nurses (QNI 2015). Initially, nursing staff were mainly working as treatment room nurses (Cartwright & Scott 1961). The 1966 contract for GPs included additional payments to cover the costs of practice staff and premises as well as the responsibility of providing 24-hour care, 365 days a year. However, this still did not really affect the work of the GPN.

In 1972 the Royal College of General Practitioners (RCGP) was created, giving GPs their own official representative body for the first time. In 1976 a three-year postgraduate training programme became mandatory for GPs. Finally, in 1978, the WHO's Alma Ata Declaration on Primary Health meant that disease prevention and health promotion increasingly started to be seen as a central part of general practice. GP practices recruiting GPNs would advertise these posts indicating that the role included a significant long-term care component, disease prevention and health promotion, and some treatment room work (such as dressings). They also offered GPNs some support to gain competencies for cervical smears, travel health and child immunisations (While & Webley-Brown 2017). However, many GPNs did not feel they received the training they were promised (While & Webley-Brown 2017).

In the 1980s the RCGP Quality Initiative was launched, in response to increasing evidence of variation in clinical practice. Early attempts to measure quality in primary care and provide incentives for improvement were met with increasing resistance. There was no significant change for GPNs until the early 1990s and the introduction of the 'internal market' (the GP fundholding system). At this point, for the first time, GPs were given budgets to commission services for their local populations. The new GP contract included chronic disease clinics and incentives to meet the population target rates for vaccinations and cervical screening. GPs therefore responded by employing nurses to provide these services (McGee & Castledine 1999). By the time this system was disbanded by the Labour government in 1998, only 33 per cent of practices were participating.

This change did, however, have a huge impact on the role of the GPN because general practice was now being seen as less curative and reactive and more preventive and proactive. The management of long-term conditions and health promotion was largely delegated to GPNs and, as a result, the numbers of nurses employed increased, as did the need for further specialised education. Research showed that, although nurses needed longer consultations for these patients, they did provide effective care (Laurant *et al.* 2005, Woodroffe 2006). A later Cochrane review (comparing GP and GPN consultations) showed that there were no consistent differences in problem recognition, examination, prescribing, and referral or diagnostic test rates or patient satisfaction (Wilson *et al.* 2006). This extended role became an important consideration when employing new staff. GPNs were also shown to offer effective services for patients with minor illnesses or ailments and those requiring same-day appointments (Shum *et al.* 2000).

Also, in the 1990s the Royal College of Nursing (RCN) Practice Nurse Forum lobbied for specialist practitioner recognition from the United Kingdom Central Council. This was achieved in 1994 (UKCC 1994) although there was not yet a recognised qualification.

Changes from 2000 to 2010

In 2004 the General Medical Services (GMS) contract was renewed and the GMS introduced the Quality and Outcomes Framework (QOF), a voluntary scheme giving GPs an incentive to provide services in addition to their core essential services. For the first time, GPs began to employ healthcare support workers or healthcare assistants (HCAs) in order to release the GPNs to focus on this specialised work. HCAs were shown to make an increasingly useful contribution to the skill mix in general practice (Bosley & Dale 2008). Not only was the HCA role reviewed, but there was a continuing incentive to educate and encourage the GPN in general practice (Sibbald, Laurant *et al.* 2006). However, it can be difficult for nurses to fulfil such a varied role when they come from a piecemeal educational background.

Alongside the changes in the contractual arrangements with general practice, there was the *2000 NHS Plan* which stated that 'the future of the NHS Plan rests on the strength of its primary care services' and this required the introduction of new models of general practice (DH 2000). In 2005 the Chief Nursing Officer introduced the *Liberating the Talents* paper which set out 10 key roles for nurses in extending and advancing their clinical roles (DH 2005). The Darzi review also encouraged the use of quality indicators at all levels in the NHS, including general practice (DH 2008). The response was the establishment of stronger regulatory and governance mechanisms, including annual appraisals for GPNs.

Changes from 2010 onwards

Within a decade, following the change from a Labour to a Conservative government, the primary care landscape had changed again – with the arrival of new Clinical Commissioning Groups (CCGs). Health Education England (HEE) and the Local Education and Training Boards (LETBs) were also formed (DH 2012a, 2012b). The Health and Social Care Act (2012) introduced comprehensive changes to the way the NHS operates, as the aim was to see more than 80,000 people with complex needs receiving community-based, GP-led, personalised care by 2014 (DH 2012b).

GPs were expected to take a lead role in independent CCGs and have greater influence over the design and delivery of local healthcare services, which included 60 per cent of the £110 billion NHS budget. The central tenet of the reforms was 'no decision about me without me' which means increasing choice and service integration, delivering care closer to home and highlighting patient involvement. This required better communication between GP practices and other services such as community nursing services, A&E, ambulance services, care homes, and mental health and social care teams (DH 2012b).

The principle that 'All UK residents are entitled by law to access primary care services, which are free at the point of need' was key to the establishment of the NHS in 1948 and was restated in the 2012 *NHS Constitution for England* (DH 2012c). Again, the workload of the nursing team increased in response to these demands. Nurses were seen to play a greater role in general practice, with the number of full-time equivalent nurses employed in general practice rising by 37 per cent between 1999 and 2006 to 14,616 (Goodwin *et al.* 2011, p. 1).

Patients' have also become more demanding in terms of what they expect from general practice; they want greater responsiveness from GP practices, better co-ordination of services and a focus on health promotion (RCGP 2007). These changing demands have led to the employment of more GPNs and HCAs. This is reflected in the fact that, between 1995 and 2008, the proportion of general practice consultations undertaken by nurses increased by 14 per cent (Hippisley Cox & Vinogradova 2009).

In 2015, in a response aimed at standardising some aspects of the nursing team training, the framework for a Care Certificate was published by Health Education England (HEE) to replace the National Minimum Training Standards (NMTS) and the Common Induction Standards (CIS) that had historically provided the framework for healthcare assistants working within health and social care.

The *Five Year Forward* plan from NHS England (2016) makes a variety of suggestions to respond to ever-changing demands in general practice. One such suggestion is that CCGs, local authorities and NHS England will be able to pool budgets to jointly commission expanded services, including the hiring of additional nurses in GP settings to provide a coordination role for patients with long-term conditions (The King's Fund 2015). It is also suggested that a GPN development strategy should include improving training capacity in general practice, increasing the number of pre-registration nurse placements, improving retention of the existing nursing workforce and supporting practice nurses to return to work (NHS England 2016).

Such a radical plan will require the investment of an additional 15 million pounds and a review of the previous piecemeal GPN training (NHS England 2016). This plan recognises the problems that will potentially occur within the next five years and mirrors the 2015 Queen's Nursing Institute report which suggested that 33.4 per cent of the GPN workforce will be due to retire by 2020 (Bradby & McCallum 2015).

> **The Queen's Nursing Institute** is a registered charity established in 1887. It is dedicated to improving the nursing care of people in the home and community. The institute has an established national network of Queen's Nurses, who are committed to the highest standards of care and who lead and inspire others. The institute also offers education grants to fund nurses to improve patient care by supporting them to develop their skills through leadership and training programmes, publishing research, influencing government, policy makers and employers, and campaigning for investment in high-quality community nursing services.
>
> *For more information go to https://www.qni.org.uk*

Box 1.1: The Queen's Nursing Institute

The 2013 HSCIC Workforce and Development Census showed that there were 23,833 GPNs, an increase of 375 (1.6 per cent) since 2012. There were also 14,943 full-time equivalent (FTE) nurses, an increase of 248 (1.7 per cent) since 2012. Although GP practices are apparently still recruiting GPNs, the level of recruitment does not reflect the scale of the need and there are concerns that they are still not recruiting many men to this career pathway. The problems with GPN recruiting may be partly due to the fact that GPN employment structure is unlike that of other community nurses, such as District Nurses or Health Visitors, where rates of pay can vary between

£14.60 and £22.00 per hour (Bradby & McCallum 2015). These long-standing issues need addressing in order to maximise GPN retention and reduce attrition (While & Webley-Brown 2017).

The QNI report also shows that many GPNs find it difficult to access ongoing education and training (Bradby & McCallum 2015). In total, 47 per cent of respondents stated that their employers did not necessarily support additional training or even offer regular appraisals. This is a real concern, bearing in mind that many GPNs have had a piecemeal journey through education to get to where they are now. In response to some of these issues, Health Education England (2015a) also launched a district nurse and general practice nursing framework developed in partnership with nursing stakeholders to standardise roles and provide a pathway to plan and develop careers. Previous frameworks were mapped against the NHS Knowledge and Skills Framework with no specific nationalised descriptions of practice nursing roles (RCGP 2012). This framework sets out the core and specific competencies and skills needed to make the change from acute to primary and community care. The main aim is to provide a much-needed career framework for GPNs, healthcare assistants (HCAs) and advanced nurse practitioners (ANPs) like the RCGP GPN Nursing Service (Fitzmaurice et al. 2015).

In 2017 Health Education England published the General Practice Workforce Development Plan in an NHS landscape awash with strategic plans and frameworks. This document was produced in response to the Five Year Forward plan and the proposed investment of at least 15 million pounds in the NHS in England (Bradby & McCallum 2015, The King's Fund 2015). Large funds were ringfenced to develop the UK's nursing workforce and this document offered clear guidance on how to increase recruitment, retention and return to practice , with examples of coherent workforce solutions for sustainable and transformational planning. Its key messages were about entry into the profession, establishing the role, enhancing it and expanding the HCA role (HEE 2017).

There are five sections in the document, with a total of 17 recommendations. The first section is about entry into general practice nursing for pre-registration nursing students and the recommendations include raising the profile of the GPN's career path, by increasing the number of pre-registration nursing placements and use of the HEE quality framework. The second section outlines recommendations for the newly qualified GPN, including strategies to increase employment of nurses on completion of their pre-registration training, preceptor programmes and GPN educator roles. The third section is about enhancing the GPN role and maximising the professional development of the workforce, by providing access to accredited training, having

GPN leaders in all CCGs and supporting nurses who wish to return to practice. The fourth section covers expanding workforce support, including the recommendation that all HCAs hold the care certificate, to increase the number of HCAs in general practice and that their training is aligned to the RCGP framework (RCGP 2012). The fifth and final section recommends a sustainable and accessible tool kit to support GPs to implement these recommendations.

The *General Practice Workforce Plan* is peppered with examples of innovative practice and delivery of educational programmes. In addition, the Queen's Nursing Institute is currently involved in a consultation process, reviewing the education and practice standards for experienced GPNs (QNI 2017b). Like all competency frameworks, these standards will seek to guide GPNs, their employers and higher education institutions in forming expectations of the role of the GPN. As GPNs, we have seen huge changes in our role and educational requirements since the 1960s. Our hope is that these reports will shape and help our profession as we move forward into the next decade. Certainly, across England, Scotland, Ireland and Wales, the GPN's role has been reviewed and several of the countries already have draft competencies for treatment nurses and GPNs in primary care. In Northern Ireland, the focus has been on reviewing:

- The scope and the developing role of GPNs within primary care
- The workforce profile within GP practices across Northern Ireland
- Recommendations on the proposed model for nursing in primary care

HSCNI (2016).

In Scotland not only were the competencies reviewed for general practice, but the Scottish government is investing £50 million pounds in order to address immediate workload and recruitment issues, as well as putting in place long-term, sustainable change within primary care; a further £10 million has been promised for mental health services (Healthcare Improvement Scotland 2016).

Other changes that may take place in the foreseeable future include developments of the GPN role from the innovative nurse apprenticeship training schemes (DH 2016, Santry 2016). There are already institutes of higher education supporting the district nurse pathway through nursing apprenticeship, so why not do the same for the GPN pathway?

Summary

In this chapter we have looked at the development of the GPN role from the early 1960s through to the present. Many aspects of the GPN role have been shaped and changed by political and economic drivers. Review what is happening in your area.

Reader activity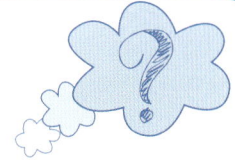

Check how much you remember about what has been discussed in this chapter. In your notebook, draw a timeline with rough dates for significant events that have influenced the development of the GPN role since the 1960s. Look back through the chapter to remind yourself of the main changes.

Box 1.2: Reader activity – timeline

Forums:

Practice Nursing forum http://www.practicenursing.co.uk/forum/forum.aspx?FORUM_ID=2

RCN General Practice Nurse Forum https://www.rcn.org.uk/get-involved/forums/general-practice-nursing-forum

Information about the role of a GPN:

Health careers – General Practice Nurse https://www.healthcareers.nhs.uk/explore-roles/nursing/general-practice-nurse

Royal College of Nursing (2014) Nurses employed by GPs: RCN guidance on good employment practice https://www.rcn.org.uk/professional-development/publications/pub-004583

Box 1.3: Resources

References

Baird, B., Charles, A., Honeyman, M., *et al.* (2016). *Understanding pressures in general practice.* London: King's Fund.

Bosley, S. & Dale, J. (2008). Healthcare assistants in general practice: practical and conceptual issues of skill-mix change. *British Journal of General Practice.* **58**(547), 118–24.

Bradby, M. & McCallum, C. (2015). *General practice nursing in the 21st century: a time of opportunity.* London: Queen's Nursing Institute.

Cartwright, A., & Scott, R. (1961). The work of a nurse employed in a general practice. *British Medical Journal.* **1**(5228), 807.

Collings, J. (1950). General practice in England today: a reconnaissance. *Lancet.* **I**, 555–85.

Department of Health (DH) (2000). *The NHS Plan.* London: HMSO.

Department of Health (DH) (2005). *Liberating the Talents.* http://webarchive.nationalarchives.gov.uk/20130107105354/http:/www.dh.gov.uk/prod_consum_dh/groups/dh_digitalassets/@dh/@en/documents/digitalasset/dh_4076250.pdf (last accessed 26.12.2018).

Department of Health (DH) (2008). *High Quality Care for All: NHS next stage review final report.* London: Department of Health.

Department of Health (DH) (2012a). *Liberating the NHS: Developing the Healthcare Workforce.* https://www.gov.uk/government/uploads/system/uploads/attachment_data/file/216421/dh_132087.pdf (last accessed 26.12.2018).

Department of Health (DH) (2012b). *Transforming Primary Care.* https://www.gov.uk/government/uploads/system/uploads/attachment_data/file/304139/Transforming_primary_care.pdf (last accessed 26.12.2018).

Department of Health (DH) (2012c). *NHS Constitution for England.* http://www.dh.gov.uk/en/Publicationsandstatistics/Publications/PublicationsPolicyAndGuidance/DH_132961 (last accessed 26.12.2018).

Fitzmaurice, D., Moger, A. & Storey, K. (2015). General practice nursing: revisited and reinvigorated. *British Journal of General Practice.* **65**(639), e636–e637.

Goodwin, N., Dixon, A.T. & Raleigh, V. (2011). *Improving the quality of care in general practice: Report of an independent inquiry commissioned by The King's Fund.* London: King's Fund. https://www.kingsfund.org.uk/sites/files/kf/improving-quality-of-care-general-practice-independent-inquiry-report-kings-fund-march-2011_0.pdf (last accessed 26.12.2018).

Health Education England (HEE) (2015a). *General practice nursing.* https://www.hee.nhs.uk/our-work/general-practice-nursing (last accessed 26.12.2018).

Health Education England (HEE) (2015b). *The Care Certificate Framework Guidance Document.* http://www.skillsforcare.org.uk/Document-library/Standards/Care-Certificate/Care-Certificate-Guidance-final---Feb-2015.pdf (last accessed 26.12.2018).

Health Education England (HEE) (2017). *The General Practice Nursing Workforce Development Plan.* https://www.hee.nhs.uk/sites/default/files/documents/The%20general%20practice%20nursing%20workforce%20development%20plan.pdf (last accessed 26.12.2018).

Healthcare Improvement Scotland (HIS) (2016). *Driving and supporting improvement in primary care: 2016–2020.* http://www.healthcareimprovementscotland.org/our_work/primary_care/programme_resources/primary_care_approach.aspx (last accessed 26.12.2018).

Health and Social Care Information Centre, (HSCIC) Workforce and Development Census (2013). HSCIC Workforce Strategy. https://medconfidential.org/wp-content/uploads/hscic/HSCIC_Board_Papers_-_05_March_2014/HSCIC131405(b)_Workforce%20Strategy%20v1.0.pdf (last accessed 5.2.2019).

Health and Social Care Northern Ireland (HSCNI) (2016). *General Practice Nursing: "Now and the Future" – A Framework for Northern Ireland.* http://www.publichealth.hscni.net/sites/default/files/General%20Practice%20Nursing%20Framework_0.pdf (last accessed 26.12.2018).

Hippisley-Cox, J. & Vinogradova, Y. (2009). *Final report to the NHS Information Centre and Department of Health Trends in consultation rates in general practice 1995/1996 to 2008/2009: Analysis of the QResearch® database.* London: NHS Information Centre for Health and Social Care.

Laurant, M., Reeves, D., Hermens, R., et al. (2005). Substitution of doctors by nurses in primary care. Cochrane Database of Systematic Reviews. April 2005. **18**(2).

McGee, P. & Castledine, G. (1999). A survey of specialised and advanced nursing practice in the UK. *British Journal of Nursing.* **8**, 1074–78.

NHS England (2014). *Five Year Forward View.* London: NHS England.

NHS England (2016). *General Practice Forward View.* https://www.england.nhs.uk/wp-content/uploads/2016/04/gpfv.pdf (last accessed 26.12.2018).

Queen's Nursing Institute (QNI) (2015). *District Nursing and General Practice Nursing Service Education and Career Framework.* https://www.hee.nhs.uk/sites/default/files/documents/Interactive%20version%20of%20the%20framework_1.pdf (last accessed 26.12.2018).

Queen's Nursing Institute (QNI) (2017a). *Transition to General Practice Nursing.* https://www.qni.org.uk/wp-content/uploads/2017/01/Transition-to-General-Practice-Nursing-CHAPTER-1.pdf (last accessed 26.12.2018).

Queen's Nursing Institute (QNI) (2017b). *General Practice Nurse Standards.* https://www.qni.org.uk/explore-qni/policy-practice/general-practice-nurse-standards/ (last accessed 26.12.2018).

Royal College of General Practitioners (RCGP) (2007). *The Future Direction of General Practice, A roadmap.* London: RCGP.

Royal College of General Practitioners (RCGP) (2012). *General Practice Nurse Competencies.* https://www.rcgp.org.uk/policy/rcgp-policy-areas/nursing.aspx (last accessed 26.12.2018).

Shum, C., Humphreys, A., Wheeler, D., Cochrane, M.A., & Clement, S. (2000). Nurse management of patients with minor illnesses in general practice: multicentre, randomised controlled trial. *British Medical Journal.* **320**(7241), 1038–43.

Sibbald, B., Laurant, M.G., & Reeves, D. (2006). Advanced nurse roles in UK primary care. *Medical Journal of Australia.* **185**(1), 10.

The King's Fund (2015). *The NHS five year forward view.* http://www.kingsfund.org.uk/projects/nhs-five-year-forward-view?gclid=CLKx6eqv7sYCFYvHtAodIhcLSA (last accessed 26.12.2018).

While, A. & Webley-Brown, C. (2017). General practice nursing: who is cherishing this workforce? *London Journal of Primary Care.* **9**(1), 10–13.

Wilson, A.D. & Childs, S. (2006). Effects of interventions aimed at changing the length of primary care physicians' consultation [review]. Cochrane Database of Systematic Reviews. 2006 (1) CD003540.

Woodroffe, E. (2006). Nurse-led general practice: the changing face of general practice? *British Journal of General Practice.* **56**(529), 632–33.

Chapter 2
Consultation skills

Deborah Duncan

Introduction

As registered nurses we adhere to *The Code* (NMC 2015 updated 2018), which sets out the values and principles we are expected to uphold and apply in a range of different practice settings. *The Code* also summarises the standards that patients and members of the public expect from health professionals and this code of conduct is a vital element in nursing. Nursing not only consists of scientific knowledge, but also encompasses interpersonal, intellectual and technical skills (Raya 2006).

The 6Cs

The NHS England 'Compassion in Practice' paper was a three-year strategy that concluded in March 2016 (NHS England 2018). The authors identified what they call the '6Cs':

- Care
- Compassion
- Competence
- Communication
- Courage
- Commitment.

These six vital elements are embedded in every aspect of nursing and midwifery and communication is one of the most important.

Communication

Communication refers to the exchange of information, thoughts and feelings between people, both verbal and non-verbal. Therapeutic communication means communication between healthcare professionals and patients and their families.

> Section 7 of the NMC Code (2018) says that nurses need to communicate clearly. To achieve this, you need to:
> - Use terms that people in your care, colleagues and the public can understand
> - Take reasonable steps to meet people's language and communication needs, providing, wherever possible, assistance to those who need help to communicate their own or other people's needs
> - Use a range of verbal and non-verbal communication methods, and consider cultural sensitivities, to better understand and respond to people's personal and health needs
> - Check people's understanding from time to time, to keep misunderstanding or mistakes to a minimum
> - Be able to communicate clearly and effectively in English.
>
> From the NMC Code (2018).

Box 2.1: The NMC Code and communication

Effective communication requires the nurse to understand the patient and what they are trying to express. This requires empathy and a patient-centred approach to care. It is also key to the provision of compassionate, high-quality nursing care (Bramhall 2014). Not only will effective communication reassure relatives that their loved ones are receiving the necessary care, but it is also considered indicative of best practice (McCabe 2004, McCabe & Timmins 2013). Certainly, the NMC (2018) Code requires nurses to 'Listen to people and respond to their preferences and concerns.'

Consultations

Most consultations end with the patient feeling satisfied, and we, as healthcare professionals, knowing that we have managed to do our job well. However, there are times when we need to break down barriers to communication to ensure that

patients feel comfortable discussing their concerns and worries (Davenport 2008). There are three aims for any effective consultation:
- To identify the patient's main problem
- To understand the patient's concerns
- To undertake a holistic assessment.

To ensure that a consultation is effective, you can use various models to help you structure the process (Kurtz & Silverman 1996, Munson & Willcox 2007). Each model has a different focus. For instance, it may take a task-orientated, patient-centred, outcomes-based or skills-based approach. The model you choose helps you to think about your consultation in a particular, structured manner. Historically, most consultation models have been produced and researched from a GP's perspective (Baird 2004). Sprague (2005) suggests that consultation models should be straightforward and practical to use. One such model is the Calgary-Cambridge model (Kurtz & Silverman 1996).

The Calgary-Cambridge model

This model is a conceptual framework (Kurtz & Silverman 1996). It was originally developed for use in medical consultations, but it is also used in nursing and by other non-medical prescriber healthcare professionals. Greenhill *et al.* (2011) list five tasks for any consultation:

A. Initiating the session

B. Gathering information

C. Building the relationship

D. Giving information – explaining and planning

E. Closing the session.

Initiating the session requires you to start by establishing a rapport with the patient. You will also want to find out why they are attending the session. Questions like 'Why have you come to see me today?' or 'I see you have booked to discuss travel vaccines – are there any other reasons why you have come?' would therefore be good ways of opening the conversation.

Once you have found out this information, you can move to part B which is **gathering information**. This section covers:
- Exploring the problems
- Understanding the patient's perspective
- Providing structure for the consultation.

Part C is **building the relationship**, which includes developing your rapport with the patient and involving them in the consultation process. The next section is **giving information or explaining and planning**. Nurses in primary care been found to carry out this task effectively, providing the type of verbal information patients require, often supplemented by written information (Seale *et al.* 2005, Venning *et al.* 2000). You also need to achieve a shared understanding, which is patient-focused, before moving on to shared decision-making and finally **closing the session**. Throughout the consultation, there should be a focus on patient-centred care, as described in the NMC Code (2018).

Pendleton's model

Pendleton's model (Pendleton *et al.* 1984) is often adapted by nurses for consultations, as it was originally written for our medical colleagues. In this model there are seven steps which, taken together, form a comprehensive and coherent list of aims for any consultation.

The first step is to identify the reason for the patient's attendance. This includes:

- The nature and history of the patient's problems
- Their aetiology
- The patient's ideas, concerns and expectations
- The effects of the problems.

The second step is to consider other related problems, including continuing problems or risk factors. The third step involves working with the patient to choose an appropriate action in response to each problem. The fourth step is the process of reaching a shared understanding of the problems with the patient. This then leads to the fifth step, which involves the patient in the management of the problem and encouraging the patient to accept appropriate responsibility. The sixth step is about using time and resources appropriately. Finally, the seventh step is to establish or maintain a relationship with the patient which helps to achieve the other tasks.

Neighbour's model (1987)

In this model there are five consultation tasks. These are defined as:

- Connecting – establishing a rapport with the patient
- Summarising – understanding why the patient has come, and summarising this back to the patient
- Handing over – includes negotiating, influencing and 'gift wrapping' (presentation of the case)

- Safety-netting – ensure a contingency plan has been made in case the patient gets worse
- Housekeeping – clearing the mind so you are ready to see the next patient.

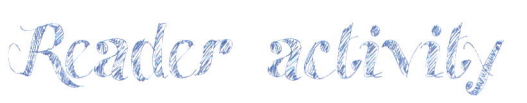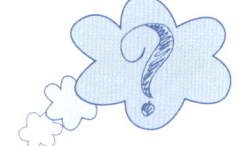

Consultation models

Spend some time with your mentor and/or reflecting on what model you will use. Then list the three main models in your notebook.

Box 2.2: Reader activity – models of consultation

Reflection

We know that reflection is a conscious effort to think about an incident that allows us to learn from it and consider how it may be enhanced, improved or done differently in the future (RCN 2018). It is also part of our revalidation process as registered nurses. Self-assessment or evaluation is part of the reflective process. We critically review the quality of our performance and our provision of nursing care and this helps us identify our strengths and weaknesses as GPNs. This process of reflection can certainly support your development and improve your consultation skills.

Patient satisfaction

Effective communication skills on the part of nurses lead to more patients feeling satisfied – because they have a clearer understanding of their diagnosis, investigations and treatment options. There is also an increased level of concordance with our clients (Maguire & Pitceathly 2002). Certainly patient-centred styles of consulting lead to an increase in patient satisfaction (Middleton 1989).

Summary

We have seen how a consultation model can help us structure our consultations. We can also see that patient satisfaction is higher in consultations when the nurse has a patient-centred approach. This is important in your role as a GPN, as so much of your role is task-focused.

References

Baird, A. (2004). Focus on... The consultation. *Nurse Prescriber.* **1**(2).

Bramhall, E. (2014). Effective communication skills in nursing practice. *Nursing Standard.* **29**(14), 53–59. doi: 10.7748/ns.29.14.53. e9355

Davenport, D. (2008). Communication – how can we improve our skills? *Nursing in Practice.* https://www.nursinginpractice.com/article/communication-how-can-we-improve-our-skills (last accessed 27.12.2018)

Greenhill, N., Anderson, C., Avery, A. & Pilnick, A. (2011). Analysis of pharmacist–patient communication using the Calgary-Cambridge guide. *Patient Education and Counseling.* **83**(3), 423–31.

Kurtz, S. & Silverman, J. (1996). The Calgary-Cambridge Referenced Observation Guides: an aid to defining the curriculum and organising teaching in communication training programmes. *Medical Education.* **30**, 838–9.

McCabe, C. (2004). Nurse–patient communication: an exploration of patients' experiences. *Journal of Clinical Nursing.* **13**(1), 41–49.

McCabe, C. & Timmins, F. (2013). *Communication Skills for Nursing Practice.* Macmillan International Higher Education.

Maguire, P. & Pitceathly, C. (2002). Key communication skills and how to acquire them. *British Medical Journal.* **325** (7366), 697–700.

Middleton, J.F. (1989). The exceptional potential of the consultation revisited. *Journal of the Royal College of General Practitioners.* **39**(326), 383–386.

Munson, E., & Willcox, A. (2007). Applying the Calgary-Cambridge model. *Practice Nursing.* **18**(9), 464–68.

Neighbour, R. (1987). *The Inner Consultation.* Lancaster: N/ITO Press.

NHS England (2016). *Making Every Contact Count (MECC): Consensus statement.* https://assets.publishing.service.gov.uk/government/uploads/system/uploads/attachment_data/file/515949/Making_Every_Contact_Count_Consensus_Statement.pdf (last accessed 27.12.2018).

NHS England (2018). *The 6cs.* https://www.england.nhs.uk/leadingchange/about/the-6cs/ (last accessed 27/12/2018).

Nursing and Midwifery Council (NMC) (2018). *The Code.* https://www.nmc.org.uk/globalassets/sitedocuments/nmc-publications/nmc-code.pdf (last accessed 27.12.2018). https://www.nmc.org.uk/globalassets/sitedocuments/nmc-publications/nmc-code.pdf (last accessed 27.12.2018).

Pendleton, D., Schofield, T., Tate, P. & Havelock, P. (1984). *The Consultation: An Approach to Learning and Teaching.* Oxford: OUP.

Ragia, A. (2006). Nursing of man as a unique person. *Nosileftiki.* **45**(1), 19–24.

Royal College of Nursing (RCN) (2018). *Revalidation requirements: Reflection and reflective discussion.* https://www.rcn.org.uk/professional-development/revalidation/reflection-and-reflective-discussion (last accessed 28.12.2018).

Seale, C., Anderson, E. & Kinnersley, P. (2005). Comparison of GP and nurse practitioner consultations: an observational study. *British Journal of General Practitioners.* **55**(521), 938–43.

Sprague, D. (2005). Consultation skills for nurse practitioners. *Independent Nurse.* VOL 6. https://www.magonlinelibrary.com/doi/full/10.12968/indn.2005.1.6.73971 (last accessed 9.4.2019)

Venning, P., Durie, A., Roland, M., Roberts, C. & Leese, B. (2000). Randomised controlled trial comparing cost effectiveness of general practitioners and nurse practitioners in primary care. *British Medical Journal.* **320**(7241), 1048–53.

Chapter 3

Public health and an introduction to health screening

Deborah Duncan

Introduction

Public health has been defined as 'the science and art of preventing disease, prolonging life and promoting health through the organised efforts of society' (Acheson 1988). Every nurse, health visitor, midwife and allied health professional can become a health-promoting practitioner (PHE 2018a). It is also what the Nursing and Midwifery Council (NMC) expects us to do, according to the Code (NMC 2018). We are encouraged to use our knowledge and skills to help improve the health and wellbeing of the public. Certainly, primary healthcare professionals are in a unique position, as gatekeepers and the first point of contact to the NHS, playing a key role in preventing illness and promoting health.

In Europe the World Health Organization (2012) suggests that the main challenges facing public health in the twenty-first century include:

- Economic crisis
- Widening inequalities
- Ageing population
- Increasing levels of chronic disease
- Migration and urbanisation
- Environmental damage and climate change.

One area causing growing concern is health inequality and how people from different economic backgrounds access healthcare (Smith & Egger 1993, Smith *et al.* 1990). This is a key aspect of the Public Health Outcomes Framework (PHE 2013).

The domains of public health

Within the Public Health Outcomes Framework (PHE 2013), the four domains are:
- Improving the wider determinants of health, which includes improving the wider factors that affect health and wellbeing, and health inequalities
- Health improvement, which involves supporting people to live healthy lifestyles, make healthy choices and reduce health inequalities
- Health protection, which includes the population's health and involves protecting the public from major incidents and other threats, while reducing health inequalities
- Healthcare public health and preventing premature mortality, which involves reducing the numbers of people living with preventable ill health and experiencing premature death and reducing the health gaps between communities.

The evidence that exists within these domains to support the public health agenda comes from national policy documents, which provide examples of practice and its effects (Marmot *et al.* 1987).

Some examples include:
- The Marmot Review
- Working Together to Safeguard Children
- Healthy Child Programme
- Every Child Matters
- Healthy Lives, Healthy People.

Public health agencies

There are public health agencies or networks across the four countries in the United Kingdom. One example is Public Health England (PHE) which is an executive agency, sponsored by the Department of Health and Social Care. PHE exists to protect and improve the nation's health and wellbeing. They also seek to reduce health inequalities.

Public Health England state that their role is to:

Make the public healthier and reduce differences between the health of different groups by promoting healthier lifestyles, advising government and supporting action by local government, the NHS and the public

Protect the nation from public health hazards such as antibiotic resistance

Prepare for and respond to public health emergencies such as an influenza epidemic

Improve the health of the whole population by sharing information and expertise, and identifying and preparing for future public health challenges

Support local authorities and the NHS to plan and provide health and social care services such as immunisation and screening programmes, and to develop the public health system and its specialist workforce

Research and analyse data to improve understanding of public health challenges and respond to public health problems such as the scarlet fever outbreak in 2018.

Adapted from PHE (2018b).

Box 3.1: The role of Public Health England

In 2016 Public Health England published its *Strategic Plan* which set out how the organisation intended to protect and improve the public's health and reduce inequalities over the next four years (PHE 2016). This led to research and work that was published in the Department of Health's *Shared Delivery Plan* (DH 2016) and the NHS *Five Year Forward View* (NHS England 2014).

The main themes were that PHE would continue to support the health and care system, building on evidence, prioritising prevention and supporting local government and the NHS. Since then PHE have certainly been active in supporting the government's legislation on standardised packs for tobacco, banning smoking in cars where children are present, trying to reduce child obesity and the sugar levy on sugary drinks. These are just a few of the challenges that public health agencies across the UK are facing.

There is a particular issue around the inequality of health outcomes between the most and least disadvantaged members of society (Marmot *et al.* 1987). People living in the most deprived communities experience poorer mental health, higher rates of smoking and greater levels of obesity than those in the more affluent areas and this difference is clearly seen in relation to the North/South economic divide.

In Northern Ireland the Public Health Agency (PHA) was established in 2009 as part of a major reform of health structures in the Island. The PHA is a multi-professional body with a strong regional and local presence. They have four key functions:

- Health and social wellbeing improvement
- Health protection
- Public health support to commissioning and policy development
- Health and social care research and development.

The stated aim of the Public Health Agency Northern Ireland is to 'protect and improve the health and social wellbeing of our population and reduce health inequalities through strong partnerships with individuals, communities and other key public, private and voluntary organisations' (PHA 2018). Their vision is much the same as that of the other three agencies: 'All people and communities are enabled and supported in achieving their full health and wellbeing potential, and inequalities in health are reduced' (PHA 2018).

In October 2016 the PHA launched a 10-year approach to transforming health and social care, supported by the Department of Health in Northern Ireland. This document *Health and Wellbeing 2026: Delivering Together* is an ambitious plan for the reform of our health and social care system. Now called the 'Delivering Together programme', it includes various work streams (DH 2018). One of these is the Community Development Work Stream, which was set up in January 2017 to examine how community development can best contribute to the Transformation Process. Again, the key driver behind this work is the need to reduce health inequalities and improve population health and wellbeing (DH 2018). It is also part of the Joint Strategic Needs Assessment, which identifies the current and future needs of the local population (PHE 2013).

Health inequalities

In many of our communities there is a social gradient in health (Nettle 2010). This means that the lower a person's social position, the worse their health is likely to be. The main factors leading to this gradient are income and work, which are two of the most important determinants of health and wellbeing. Although unemployment has been falling in England, the percentage of unemployed people increases for those living in the most deprived areas and is more than double that of the least deprived areas (PHE 2017). Unemployment affects both mental and physical health outcomes.

Nettle (2010) suggests that people in the lower socioeconomic groups tend to smoke more, exercise less, have less healthy diets, have poor concordance with therapy, utilise medical services less, do not act on health and safety advice and are generally less health-conscious than their more affluent peers. Certainly, those who live in deprived areas experience the worst health outcomes, with increased morbidity and mortality (Lynch *et al.* 2000).

In Northern Ireland, around 23 per cent of children are reported to be living in poverty (Rowntree 2018). There are inequalities in life expectancy, in young men, ethnic minorities, migrants, carers, lesbian, gay, bisexual and transgender people, the homeless populations and those with a disability.

In Wales the public health agency, Public Health Wales, is accountable to the seven Health Boards responsible for delivering all healthcare services in specified geographical areas (NHS Wales 2018). Their responsibilities of Public Health Wales are outlined in Box 3.2 (below).

The responsibilities of Public Health Wales are:
- Investigation and management of all communicable diseases
- Surveillance of communicable diseases
- Development of the immunisation strategy, as well as supporting and monitoring immunisation programmes
- Advising on community infection control
- Dissemination of information on communicable diseases to community
- Advising on environmental health issues
- Dealing with health protection queries from all agencies
- Facilitating the completion of the LHB audits of child protection
- Involvement in child protection case reviews
- Advising on 'Out of County placements'
- Child training for NHS Boards
- Providing specialist dental public health advice to improve oral health, support planning of dental services and ensure patient safety for dental patients.

Box 3.2: The responsibilities of Public Health Wales
(Public Health Wales 2017, NHS Wales 2018)

In Scotland there is a Scottish public health network (The ScotPHN), hosted by NHS Health Scotland, which is accountable to the Scottish Directors of Public Health. It is open to anyone with a professional interest and involvement in the wider health improvement agenda. In June 2018 NHS Scotland published Public Health Priorities for Scotland.

It has been recognised that overall health in Scotland is unacceptably poor, compared to other Western European countries (NHS Scotland 2018). Many people living in the most deprived communities still experience poorer health than those living in our wealthier areas (NHS Scotland 2018). Again, the need to tackle the health inequalities that prevent good health is therefore high on the agenda (NHS Scotland 2018). Now we have looked at the public health agencies across the UK, please spend some time looking at the next reader activity in Box 3.3 (below).

Reader activity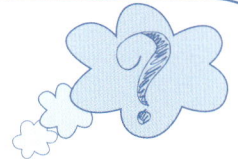

What are the major national policy documents relating to your area of practice? These may be local or regional. Look at the public health organisation website for your region.

Public Health England: https://www.gov.uk/government/organisations/public-health-england

Public Health Wales: http://www.publichealthwales.wales.nhs.uk/

Public Health Scotland: http://www.healthscotland.com/resources/networks/scotphn/about.aspx

Public Health Northern Ireland: http://www.publichealth.hscni.net/

Box 3.3: Reader activity – policy documents

Models of health promotion

There are several theories and models that support the practice of health promotion and disease prevention. You should have covered these in your pre-registration training. This section will give you a refresher. These theories are used in the development of local and national educational programmes and are often related to behavioural change. The four key models used in public health interventions are: the Health Belief Model, the Transtheoretical or Stages of Change Model, Social Cognitive Theory and the Social Ecological Models.

The Health Belief Model (HBM), developed in the 1950s, was one of the first theories of health behaviour. It focuses on addressing problem behaviours that cause health concerns such as high-risk sexual behaviour and the possibility of contracting HIV (Croyle 2005). This model proposes that a person's health-related behaviour depends on their perception of four critical areas:

- The severity of a potential illness
- The person's susceptibility to that illness
- The benefits of taking a preventive action
- The barriers to taking that action.

It suggests that people engage or disengage in health-promoting behaviour according to their beliefs about health problems, the perceived benefits of action and barriers to action, and their own self-efficacy (Janz *et al.* 1984).

The Transtheoretical Model (TTM) is also called the Stages of Change Model. This was developed by Prochaska and DiClemente in the late 1970s, looking at the experiences of smokers – who quit and why (Prochaska & DiClemente 2005: precontemplation, contemplation, preparation, action, maintenance and termination. For each stage of change, there are different intervention strategies.

Social Cognitive Theory considers what health promotion and disease prevention are, and looks at the causal structures that affect behaviour and behavioural outcomes. It considers such factors as people's self-efficacy beliefs, their outcome expectations and environmental factors and how these influence human behaviour and well-being (Bandura 2004).

The Social Ecological Models consider the interactive characteristics of individuals and environments that affect health outcomes. They were first discussed by sociologists associated with the Chicago School after the First World War. They focus on links between behavioural theories and anthropology.

Making Every Contact Count

NHS Health Education England have also launched an initiative called 'Making Every Contact Count' (NHS HEE). This is an approach to behaviour change that utilises everyday interactions with other people to support them in making positive changes to their physical and mental health and wellbeing, as many long-term diseases are closely linked to behavioural factors (Newton *et al.* 2015). This framework is obviously part of the consultation process but also considers the 'millions of day-to-day interactions that organisations and people have with other people' (PHE 2016). The message consists of concise healthy lifestyle information that you would use in a brief intervention.

Health literacy

Health literacy is another important aspect of health promotion. This is defined as 'the degree to which individuals have the cognitive and social skills to appropriately access, understand and use health information and services to maintain good health' (Paasche-Orlow *et al.* 2005). Poor health literacy is linked with poor health and health outcomes such as reduced self-management capacity (Berkman *et al.* 2011). Therefore, improving health literacy is important in order to improve people's ability to care for themselves. What initiatives have been taken in your local area to improve health literacy?

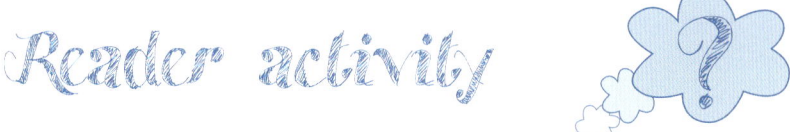

Identify the four key theories used in health promotion, then discuss them with your mentor.

Box 3.4: Reader activity – health promotion theory (answers on p. 25)

Summary

As we have seen, health promotion and disease prevention are key government priorities. We should also remember that GPNs have a unique role within healthcare practices, in terms of engaging with the wider public health agenda, as they are often the patient's first point of contact with the NHS. An understanding of the different theories used in health promotion is also helpful in any public health involvement.

> **Reader activity**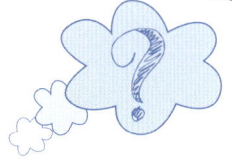
>
> Define the four key theories used in health promotion:
> - Health Belief Model
> - The Transtheoretical Model and Stages of Change
> - Social Cognitive Theory
> - Social Ecological Model

Box 3.5: Answers to reader activity – health promotion theory

References

Acheson, D. (1988). *Public Health in England: The Report of the Committee of Inquiry into the Future Development of the Public Health Function*. London: HMSO.

Bandura, A. (2004). Health Promotion by Social Cognitive Means. *Health Education & Behavior.* **31**(2), 143–64.

Berkman, N.D., Sheridan, S.L., Donahue, K.E., Halpern, D.J. & Crotty, K. (2011). Low health literacy and health outcomes: An updated systematic review. *Annals of Internal Medicine.* **155**(2), 97.

Croyle, R.T. (2005). *Theory at a Glance: Application to Health Promotion and Health Behaviour.* 2nd ed. Department of Health and Human Services, National Institutes of Health.
Available at https://www.thecommunityguide.org/ (last accessed 31.12.2018).

Department of Health and Social Care (2018). *Expansion of Community Development Approaches: Report to Transformation Implementation Group.* http://www.publichealth.hscni.net/sites/default/files/Expansion%20of%20Community%20Development%20Approaches%20Report%20-%202018%20May%202018%20MB.pdf (last accessed 31.12.2018).

Janz, Nancy K. & Marshall H. Becker (1984). The Health Belief Model: A decade later. *Health Education & Behavior.* **11**(1), 1–47. doi:10.1177/109019818401100101.

Lynch, J.W., Davey Smith, G., Kaplan, G.A. & House, J.S. (2000). Income inequality and mortality: importance to health of individual income, psychosocial environment, or material conditions. *British Medical Journal.* **320**, 1200–1204.

Marmot, M.G., Kogevinas, M. & Elston, M.A. (1987). Social-economic status and disease. *Annual Review of Public Health.* **8**, 111–35.

Nettle, D. (2010). Why are there social gradients in preventative health behavior? A perspective from behavioral ecology. *PLOS One.*
https://doi.org/10.1371/journal.pone.0013371 (last accessed 31.12.2018).

Newton, J.N., Briggs, A.D., Murray, C.J. (2015). Changes in health in England, with analysis by English regions and areas of deprivation, 1990–2013: a systematic analysis for the Global Burden of Disease Study 2013; Public Health England. *Lancet.* **386**, 2257–74.

NHS Health Education England (2018). *Making Every Contact Count.*
http://www.makingeverycontactcount.co.uk/ (last accessed 31.12.2018).

NHS Wales (2018). *Local Public Health.*
http://www.wales.nhs.uk/sitesplus/888/home (last accessed 5.2.2019).

NHS Scotland (2018). *Public Health Priorities for Scotland.*
http://www.gov.scot/Resource/0053/00536757.pdf (last accessed 31.12.2018).

Nursing and Midwifery Council (NMC) (2018). *The Code.* https://www.nmc.org.uk/globalassets/sitedocuments/nmc-publications/nmc-code.pdf (last accessed 27.12.2018).

Paasche-Orlow, M.K., Parker, R.M., Gazmararian, J.A., Nielsen-Bohlman, L T. & Rudd, R.R. (2005). The prevalence of limited health literacy. *Journal of General Internal Medicine.* **20**(2), 175–84.

Public Health Agency (PHA) (2018). *About us.*
http://www.publichealth.hscni.net/about-us (last accessed 31.12.2018).

Prochaska, J. & DiClemente, Carlo C. (2005). 'The transtheoretical approach'. In Norcross, John C., Goldfried & Marvin R. (eds) *Handbook of psychotherapy integration.* Oxford series in clinical psychology (2nd ed.). Oxford & New York: Oxford University Press. pp. 147–71.

Public Health England (PHE) (2013). *The evidence base of the public health contribution of nurses and midwives.* https://assets.publishing.service.gov.uk/government/uploads/system/uploads/attachment_data/file/208842/Evidence.pdf (last accessed 31.12.2018).

Public Health England (PHE) (2016). *Strategic plan for the next four years: Better outcomes by 2020.* https://assets.publishing.service.gov.uk/government/uploads/system/uploads/attachment_data/file/516985/PHE_Strategic_plan_2016.pdf (last accessed 31.12.2018).

Public Health England (PHE) (2017). *Research and analysis.* Chapter 6: social determinants of health. https://www.gov.uk/government/publications/health-profile-for-england/chapter-6-social-determinants-of-health#main-messages (last accessed 31.12.2018).

Public Health England (PHE) (2018a). *Tools and models to support the development of the public health contribution of nurses, midwives and allied health professionals.*
https://www.gov.uk/government/collections/developing-the-public-health-contribution-of-nurses-and-midwives-tools-and-models (last accessed 31.12.2018).

Public Health England (PHE) (2018b). *About us.*
https://www.gov.uk/government/organisations/public-health-england/about (last accessed 31.12.2018).

Public Health Wales (2017). *Our Strategic Plan 2017–20.*
http://www.wales.nhs.uk/sitesplus/documents/888/Integrated%20Medium%20Term%20Plan%202017-2020%20v1.pdf (last accessed 31.12.2018).

Rowntree, J. (2018). *Poverty in Northern Ireland.*
https://www.jrf.org.uk/report/poverty-northern-ireland-2018 (last accessed 31.12.2018).

Smith, G.D. & Egger, M. (1993). Socioeconomic differentials in wealth and health. *British Medical Journal.* **307**, 1085–86.

Smith, G.D., Bartley, M. & Blane, D. (1990). The Black report on socioeconomic inequalities in health 10 years on. *British Medical Journal.* **301**, 373–377.

Virtanen, P., Kivimaki, M., Vahtera, J. & Koskenvuo, M. (2006). Employment status and differences in the one-year coverage of physician visits: different needs or unequal access to services? BMC Health Services Research 6.

World Health Organisation (WHO) (2012). *European Action Plan for Strengthening Public Health Capacities and Services.* http://www.euro.who.int/__data/assets/pdf_file/0005/171770/RC62wd12rev1-Eng.pdf?ua=1 (last accessed 31.12.2018).

Chapter 4

Cervical cytology

Sian Hayes and Deborah Duncan

Introduction

The NHS Cervical Screening Programme (NHSCSP) has been running since the 1960s in the United Kingdom. It was initially just designed for cervical screening but in the late 1980s it incorporated computing systems that provided an automated call and recall system and a central records agency. In 2004 liquid-based cytology was introduced, as this has been found to significantly reduce the number of inadequate smears. Other important campaigns have included the identification of the human papilloma virus (HPV) and its relation to cervical cancer, and the introduction of the vaccination programme in 2008 for all girls aged 12 to 13 (NHS Choices 2018).

Cervical screening

The aim of the NHSCSP is to reduce the number of people who develop invasive cervical cancer and those who die from it. The programme offers regular screening to eligible individuals in order to identify and treat those conditions which have the potential to develop into invasive cancer.

Like any screening programme, it meets the ten screening criteria devised by Wilson & Jungner (1968) for the World Health Organisation:

1. The condition sought should be an important health problem
2. There should be an accepted treatment for patients with recognised disease
3. Facilities for diagnosis and treatment should be available

4. There should be a recognisable latent or early symptomatic stage
5. There should be a suitable test or examination
6. The test should be acceptable to the population
7. The natural history of the condition, including development from latent to declared disease, should be adequately understood
8. There should be an agreed policy on whom to treat as patients
9. The cost of case finding (including diagnosis and treatment of patients diagnosed) should be economically balanced in relation to possible expenditure on medical care as a whole
10. Case finding should be a continuing process and not a 'once and for all' project.

Cervical cytology screening meets these criteria and it is clearly a beneficial programme which saves lives, as it helps prevents the development of cervical cancer. Women have a cervical smear taken, in which a sample of cells is taken from their cervix. Using liquid-based cytology (LBC), these samples are sent to a local laboratory, which examines them under the microscope to look for any abnormal changes in the cells. The results are forwarded to the service users and are also held on a national database.

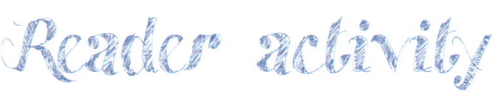 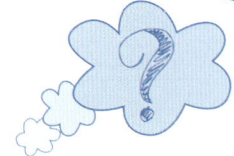

In your notebook, draw a timeline with dates relating to significant events in the development of the NHS Cervical Screening Programme (NHSCSP).

Box 4.1: Reader activity – timeline

Epidemiology

Cancer of the cervix is the second most common cancer among women worldwide and approximately 80 per cent of cases occur in developing countries, which equates to more than 265,000 women dying from cervical cancer in 2012 worldwide. It is also the twelfth most common cause of cancer deaths in women in the UK; in 2013 that meant over 3200 women were diagnosed with cervical cancer.

The success of the cervical screening programme is shown by the fact that deaths from cervical cancer have fallen in England by over 70 per cent since the early 1970s. It is therefore estimated that cervical screening saves 4500 lives per year in England (NCRAS

2016). Updated evidence from the Joint Committee on Vaccination and Immunisation (JCVI) recommends that the existing HPV vaccination programme for girls should be extended to boys as well. Pilot areas are now vaccinating boys aged between 12 and 13 in England (GOV 2018). This decision follows new scientific evidence and advice from an independent panel of experts. Nevertheless, cervical screening coverage in England is at a 21-year low, down from 72 per cent in 2017 and 73.7 per cent in 2011 (Music 2018).

Human papilloma virus (HPV)

The human papilloma virus (HPV) causes an infection which can present in different ways. In most cases the infection causes no symptoms and can resolve spontaneously; in other patients it presents with warts of the mouth, throat, penis or anus. It can, however, lead to precancerous lesions that can increase the risk of cancer of the cervix and other cancers of the genito-urinary system. There are over 200 types of the virus, approximately 40 of which are transmitted through sexual contact. Approximately 70 per cent of all cervical cancer is due to HPV types 16 and 18 (WHO 2016).

Ages for screening

Women are invited to attend for screening when they reach the age of 25. This is because HPV infection is less likely to persist in younger women. Many have low-grade abnormalities which revert to normal with time (Sasieni *et al.* 2010). The incidence of cervical cancer in those under 25 years of age is very low (Sasieni *et al.* 2009). A woman's first invitation to attend routine cervical screening should be sent out six months before her 25th birthday. This is because a delay of several months may occur between the issuing of invitations to women and the date of their screening test (Richardson *et al.* 2007).

Recommended screening intervals

Age	Frequency of screening
24.5	First invitation
25 to 49	Three-yearly
50 to 64	Five-yearly
65+	Invitations as required for women who have had recent abnormal tests. Women who have not had an adequate screening test reported since age 50 may be screened on request.

Box 4.2: Screening ages

Screening is stopped for women at the age of 65, as the prevalence of severely abnormal cells found on the surface of the cervix, known as high-grade or severe dysplasia (or CIN 3), and invasive cancer, is low in women over the age of 50 (PHE 2016a).

If women outside the screening age experience vaginal bleeding after sex and/or in between periods, they require a pelvic examination. It is important to note that vaginal bleeding is extremely common and can be due to cervical ectropion, hormonal changes, benign cervical polyps or sexually transmitted infections. However, the underlying cause does need to be identified (NHS 2010).

People eligible for screening

Transgender men

People who are transgender (trans) men, who still have a cervix, are eligible for screening. If they are registered with their GP under a female gender, they will automatically be sent a screening invitation. Trans men who are registered as male won't get an invitation but do remain entitled to screening. However, they will only know if we advertise this service to patients, their families and their support groups.

Women who are not sexually active

All women between the ages of 25 and 64 are eligible for cervical screening but if the women have never been sexually active they have a low chance of developing cervical cancer. These women are considered to be at 'no or very low risk' and they often decline the usual screening invitation.

Call and recall

One of the fundamental principles of any screening programme is to ensure that all the individuals who are eligible for screening receive the appropriate invitations to participate at the correct time. This administrative process is often referred to as the 'call and recall' system. In the UK there is a nationally recognised service called Open Exeter that supports this service. It is a web-enabled viewer which has a facility to share information held on the DMS (NHAIS) database. Open Exeter also holds details of women's cervical screening history, including the date, the result and the recommendation made by the laboratory for recall interval (NHS England 2015). Each GP practice will have a nominated person who can access Open Exeter and is responsible for call and recall.

The call and recall system includes the method of generating the lists of women who are due to be invited for cervical screening. It also includes the system to send out letters and reminders, to record the test results and forward them to the women.

Voluntary withdrawal from screening

Women can withdraw from the cervical cytology programme by written request. Reasons can vary from being at low risk of cervical cancer to having a physical or learning disability which makes sample taking difficult (PHE 2016).

HPV triage and test of cure
HPV triage
With the new high-risk human papilloma virus (HR-HPV) triage, women whose cervical samples show borderline changes are tested for HPV. Those with HPV-positive results are automatically referred for colposcopy. Those with a negative HPV test result are returned to routine recall (PHE 2016a).

HPV test of cure
HPV test of cure (TOC) uses HR-HPV testing to assess women who have already received treatment for cervical intra-epithelial neoplasia (CIN) and cervical glandular intra-epithelial neoplasia (CGIN). Healthcare professionals can use a TOC pathway to decide if the woman needs a referral for further assessment or if she can slot back into the three-yearly recall.

Taking a smear

It is important to note that clinicians performing cervical screening are trained in accordance with local and national guidelines. Not only do they have to receive training on a recognised course but they also undertake a minimum of one half-day update training every three years. These guidelines are outlined by Public Health England in their publication NHS Cervical Screening Programme Guidance for the training of cervical sample takers (PHE 2016b). This ensures that smear takers meet the clinical governance requirements. Women themselves will also feel confident in the screening programme. They expect a trained and competent professional who can offer the appropriate communication, empathy, skill and reassurance during this intimate examination (PHE 2016b).

The Royal College of Nursing provides the following best practice guidelines for taking a smear (RCN 2013):

- Establish a rapport with the patient. You will also need to gain their consent for this intimate procedure.
- Check that they are currently eligible for a smear and answer any questions they may have.

- Ensure you have filled in the correct paperwork.
- Check that you have all the equipment you will need. You will need to use the correct procedure for your local guidelines and liquid-based cytology method. You will need an adjustable couch, an adjustable light source, a trolley with appropriately sized speculum, sampling device and gloves and an appropriately labelled vial.
- Ask the patient if they need to empty their bladder.
- Check whether they want a chaperone or not, as all patients are entitled to have one (RCN 2002). They will need to strip from the waist down.
- Ask them to lie on the bed with their ankles together and allow their knees to spread apart as much as possible.
- Wash your hands and put on some gloves.
- Talking to the patient and explaining what you are doing, inspect the vagina for any abnormalities. Ensure the speculum has been lubricated with warm water or a recommended gel. It is important to follow local guidelines, as the wrong lubricant can cause problems with the delicate laboratory equipment used to screen the samples.
- The next step is to use your left hand to part the labia minora and insert the speculum with the screw facing sideways.
- Open the blades approximately 5mm and gently and seamlessly guide the speculum until the anterior lip of the cervix can be seen.
- Then open the speculum to expose the cervix.
- As you insert the speculum, turn it so that the screw faces upwards and then open the blades and fix them open with the screw. You may need to adjust your light source.
- Identify the cervix and the transformation zone.
- Inspect the cervix, looking at its appearance and colour. Note any secretions. Report your findings and explain them to your patient.
- Obtain the sample using the appropriate sampling tool. Again, inform the woman about what you are doing.
- Place the sample in the liquid-based cytology vial as per instructions.
- Then slowly remove the speculum from vagina.

After the smear test it is important to remind the woman how and when she will receive her results.

Cervical cytology

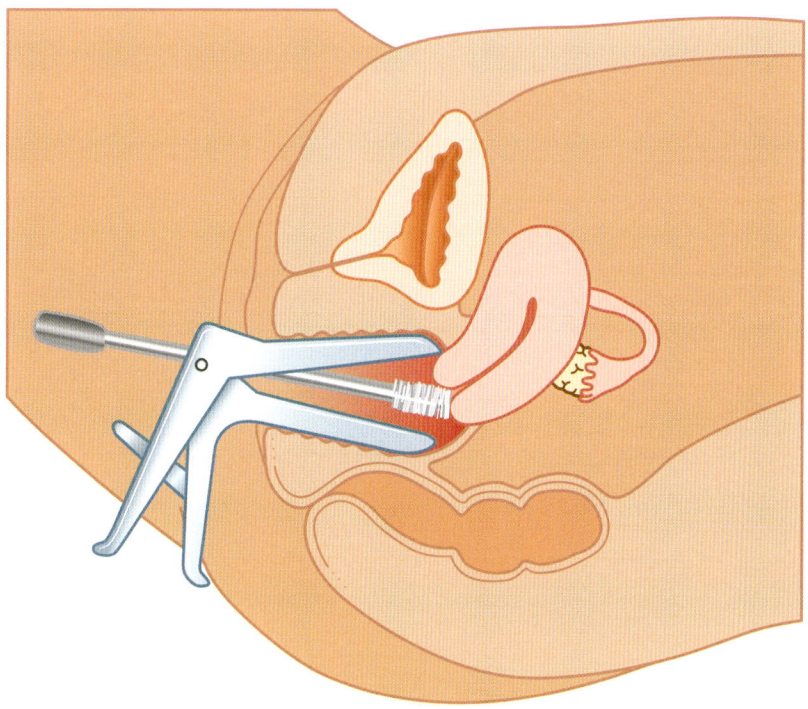

Figure 4.1: Taking a smear (Getty Images)

Summary

Cervical cytology is an important aspect of the NHSCSP. It is also a core aspect of the GPN's role. As part of your foundational training, you will be expected to complete nationally accredited cervical cytology training. This chapter will support you in your training and it is also important that you attend regular updates.

References

GOV (2018). HPV vaccine to be given to boys in England. https://www.gov.uk/government/news/hpv-vaccine-to-be-given-to-boys-in-england (last accessed 23.1.2019).

Joint Committee on Vaccination and Immunisation (JCVI) (2017). JCVI Interim Statement on Extending HPV Vaccination to Adolescent Boys. https://assets.publishing.service.gov.uk/government/uploads/system/uploads/attachment_data/file/630125/Extending_HPV_Vaccination.pdf (last accessed 1.1.2019).

Music, R. (2018). *Falling cervical screening attendance in England could cost lives.* https://www.jostrust.org.uk/node/1075999 (last accessed 1.1.2019).

National Cancer Registration and Analysis Service (NCRAS) (2016). http://www.ncin.org.uk/publications/reports/ (last accessed 1.1.2019).

NHS (2010). *Clinical Practice Guidance for the Assessment of Young Women aged 20–24 with Abnormal Vaginal Bleeding.* https://www.gov.uk/government/uploads/system/uploads/attachment_data/file/436924/doh-guidelines-young-women.pdf (last accessed 1.1.2019).

NHS Choices (2018). *Overview: Cervical screening.* https://www.nhs.uk/conditions/cervical-screening/ (last accessed 1.1.2019).

NHS England (2015). *DMS Medical Centre Guide to using Open Exeter for Cervical Screening Call/Recall.* https://www.england.nhs.uk/commissioning/wp-content/uploads/sites/12/2015/05/f-dms-med-centre-oe-guide.pdf (last accessed 1.1.2019).

Public Health England (PHE) (2016a). *NHS Cervical Screening Programme. Colposcopy and Programme Management NHSCSP Publication number 20.* https://www.bsccp.org.uk/assets/file/uploads/resources/NHSCSP_20_Colposcopy_and_Programme_Management_(3rd_Edition)_(2).pdf (last accessed 1.1.2019).

Public Health England (PHE) (2016b). *NHS Cervical Screening Programme Guidance for the training of cervical sample takers.* https://www.gov.uk/government/uploads/system/uploads/attachment_data/file/577158/NHS_Cervical_Screening_Progamme_-_guidance_for_cervical_sample_takers.pdf (last accessed 1.1.2019).

Royal College of Nursing (RCN) (2002). *RCN's guidance for nursing staff. Chaperoning: the role of the nurse and rights of patients.* Available from libraries.

Royal College of Nursing (RCN) (2013). *Cervical Screening.* https://www.rcn.org.uk/professional-development/publications/pub-003105 (last accessed 1.1.2019).

Richardson, J., Howe, A. & McElduff, P. (2007). *Time Dependent Response to Invitation for Cervical Screening* (NHSCSP Publication No 29). Sheffield: NHS Cancer Screening Programmes. http://www.cancerscreening.nhs.uk/cervical/publications/nhscsp20.pdf (last accessed 9.4.2019).

Sasieni, P., Castanon, A. & Cuzick J. (2010). *Impact of cervical screening on young women: a critical review of the literature* (NHSCSP Publication No 31). Sheffield: NHS Cancer Screening Programmes. https://www.cervicalcheck.ie/_fileupload/Image/The_Impact_of_Cervical_Screening_on_Young_Women_02406561.pdf (last accessed 1.1.2019).

Sasieni, P., Castanon, A. & Cuzick J. (2009). Effectiveness of cervical screening with age: Population based case-control study of prospectively recorded data. *British Medical Journal.* **339**, b2968.

Wilson, J.M.G. & Jungner, G. (1968). *Principles and practice of screening for disease.* Geneva: WHO. http://apps.who.int/iris/bitstream/handle/10665/37650/WHO_PHP_34.pdf?sequence=17 (last accessed 1.1.2019).

World Health Organisation (WHO) (2016). *Human papillomavirus (HPV) and cervical cancer.* http://www.who.int/mediacentre/factsheets/fs380/en/ (last accessed 1.1.2019).

Chapter 5

Women's health

Deborah Duncan

Introduction

Women's health is a very broad subject and GPNs mainly focus on family planning, prevention and screening programmes (such as cervical cytology and breast screening).

When we consider women's health, common questions may include:

- What causes bleeding between periods?
- How should I check my breasts?
- What are pelvic floor exercises?
- What is a well woman clinic?
- Do I need a cervical screening test if I'm a virgin?

The World Health Organisation defines health as 'a state of complete physical, mental and social well-being and not merely the absence of disease or infirmity' (WHO, n.d.). In the case of women, this focuses on reproductive and sexual health.

The usual menstrual cycle

It is helpful to be reminded of the normal menstrual cycle when we think of women's health. It is an important aspect of education in family planning and identification of disease. As clinicians, we need to be able to differentiate between normal and abnormal menstruation. The average age of menarche is approximately 12.5 years of age. The usual end of the menstrual cycles is called the menopause and it normally occurs between 45 and 55 years of age.

The usual menstrual cycle begins on the first day of bleeding and is counted as day one. The cycle ends just before the next menstrual period and can therefore range from about 25 to 36 days. It is estimated that only 10 to 15 per cent of women have cycles that are exactly 28 days; 20 per cent of women have irregular cycles that are normal for them. In fact Munster *et al.* (1992) found that 29.3 per cent of all women had a menstrual cycle with a variation of >14 days. They suggested that definitions of polymenorrhoea (cycle length <21 days) and oligomenorrhoea (cycle length between 36 and 90 days) were commonly used but that this high percentage of women with an abnormal cycle challenges the view that a variation >5 days should be regarded as a sign of disease in the woman (Munster *et al.* 1992). In fact, a later study by Fehring *et al.* (2006) showed that 95 per cent of the cycles were between 22 and 36 days. There are various factors that can lead to an irregular cycle, including obesity and polycystic ovary syndrome (Wei *et al.* 2009).

Normal menstrual bleeding lasts 3 to 7 days with the average being 5 days. The blood loss during a cycle usually ranges from ½ to 2 ½ ounces. Irregular cycles, or irregular periods, is an abnormal variation in the usual length of a woman's menstrual cycle. A variation of 21 days or more is considered very irregular (Kippley & Kipplcy 1996). There can also be a change in the menstrual cycle due to the circadian rhythms by sleep disturbances or altered melatonin production (Lawson *et al.* 2011).

Hormones of the menstrual cycle

The menstrual cycle is regulated by luteinizing hormone and follicle-stimulating hormone, which are produced by the pituitary gland. Gaining a clear understanding of these hormones will help you understand the way hormonal contraception works.

There are three phases within the normal menstrual or ovarian cycle. These are:
- The follicular stage (before the release of the egg)
- The ovulatory stage (when the egg is released)
- The luteal stage (after the egg is released).

The uterine cycle is divided into:
- Menstruation
- The proliferative phase
- The secretory phase.

Ovulation generally occurs as early as the eighth day of the cycle and as late as the 60th day of the menstrual cycle (Wilcox *et al.* 2006). Normal ovulation occurs every 21–35 days between the time of menarche and menopause.

During the follicular phase, there is an increasing amount of oestrogen, which causes the blood or menses to stop and the lining of the uterus thickens ready for implantation of the fertilised egg. The follicles in the ovary develop, affected by the hormones, so that one or two develop to maturity.

At midcycle ovulation occurs, 24–36 hours after the luteinizing hormone level surges and the dominant follicle releases an oocyte or egg. The remains of the follicle develop into the corpus luteum, which is released. Progesterone causes the uterine lining to prepare for the potential implantation of an embryo.

If implantation does not occur within two weeks, the corpus luteum will fail, resulting in a drop of progesterone and oestrogen, followed by the shedding of the uterine lining.

Progesterone-only contraception

Progestogen-only contraceptives decrease the gonadotropin-releasing hormone (GnRH) released by the hypothalamus. This in turn decreases the release of follicle-stimulating hormone (FSH) and luteinizing hormone (LH) by the anterior pituitary. A reduction of FSH inhibits the follicular development and the rise in oestradiol levels.

Combined hormonal contraceptives

Combined oral contraceptives contain both an oestrogen and a progestogen hormone acting on the menstrual cycle. There is a decrease in the release of FSH and follicular development, preventing ovulation.

These combined hormonal contraceptives are effective because:
- They are reliable and reversible
- They are an effective treatment for dysmenorrhoea and menorrhagia
- They reduce the incidence of premenstrual tension
- Women are found to have less benign breast disease
- There is a reduced risk of ovarian and endometrial cancer
- There is a reduced risk of pelvic inflammatory disease.

NICE (2018).

Contraception and the family planning service

The first birth control clinic in the UK was opened in London in 1921 by Marie Stopes. Then, between 1921 and 1930, five different birth control societies were formed, which were later amalgamated to form the National Birth Control Council in the 1930s. At that time the Ministry of Health permitted local health authorities (LHAs) to provide birth control advice only for married women if pregnancy would be detrimental to their health.

Reader activity

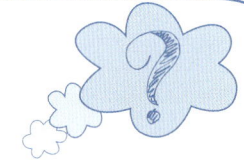

Find out what you can about the following methods of contraception. Also discuss with your mentor where patients can access these types of contraception in your local area:
- Caps or diaphragms
- Combined pill
- Condoms
- Contraceptive implant
- Contraceptive injection
- Contraceptive patch
- Female condoms
- IUD (intrauterine device or coil)
- IUS (intrauterine system or hormonal coil)
- Natural family planning (fertility awareness)
- Progestogen-only pill
- Vaginal ring.

Also look at the two permanent methods of contraception:
- Female sterilisation
- Male sterilisation (vasectomy).

Box 5.1: Reader activity – types of contraception (answers on p. 42)

It wasn't until 1967 that the National Health Service (Family Planning) Act enabled LHAs to give birth control advice, regardless of marital status. In 1968 Section 15 of the Health Services and Public Health Act 1968 allowed the same amendments in Scotland. Then, in 1972, the National Health Service (Family Planning) Amendment Act empowered local health authorities to offer free vasectomies for men and in April of that same year all contraceptive advice and prescribed supplies provided by the NHS became free of charge irrespective of the patient's age or marital status. In 1977 the National Health Service Act charged the Secretary of State with ensuring that the full range of contraceptive services was available and free of charge.

Since then there have been a great number of changes in this provision, from the 1984 DHSS guidelines on provision of contraceptives to under-16s and Gillick competency to ongoing cuts in the NHS. In the early 2000s primary care trusts became responsible for planning and securing the provision of local healthcare and services. Alongside these changes was the development of the extended role of the nurse in prescribing. From 2004, independent nurse prescribers were able to prescribe from the full formulary.

Since then, we have seen the development of non-medical prescribing, allowing practical changes to our family planning services. There are also regional differences to these services in the UK. In Northern Ireland women cannot access services for termination. In response to changes in abortion law in the South of Ireland, the UK government announced that women travelling from Northern Ireland to England would no longer be charged to access abortion services. This will eventually extend to accommodation costs too. Furthermore, in March 2018 a central booking system provided by the British Pregnancy Advisory Service was established, to support women travelling from Northern Ireland to access abortion services in England.

Contraception is still free from the NHS, though it can be confusing to access . Generally, these services are offered through local GP surgeries, sexual health clinics and local pharmacies.

Female genital mutilation (FGM)

Female genital mutilation (FGM) refers to procedures that intentionally alter or cause injury to the female genital organs (WHO 2018b). This procedure is carried out for non- medical reasons and has no health benefits for the patient. FGM is a violation of human rights (WHO 2018b). Find out what training provision is available in your area on FGM, which is currently receiving a lot of attention from the Department of Health.

Long-term medical conditions and women

Some long-term conditions are more prevalent in women. For instance, there is a higher cardiovascular risk and diabetes is more prevalent among women with polycystic ovary syndrome (Wild *et al.* 2000). The underlying cause of the higher incidence of some long-term conditions in women is unknown. However, we do know that women tend to smoke for longer periods than men and are therefore at greater risk from the effects of smoking (Huisman *et al.* 2005). The long-term cumulative effect of pack-years of smoking in women is likely to increase the rate of COPD in the UK (Soriano *et al.* 2000).

Cancer and women

Lung cancer is the leading cause of cancer death in women, followed by breast cancer, colorectal, ovarian, uterine and cervical cancers. However, breast cancer is the most common cancer in women in developed countries. Each year, 1200 women are diagnosed with breast cancer, with 55,122 having invasive breast cancer (Cancer Research UK 2018). Around 23 per cent of these cases are preventable through early detection and screening (Cancer Research UK 2018, IBSR 2012). Although breast cancer is usually seen in women who are over 50 years of age and who have reached menopause, any woman can get it (IBSR 2012). It is also found in men.

Breast screening

As the risk of developing breast cancer increases with age, all women aged 50 to 70 are automatically invited for breast cancer screening (mammograms) every three years via their GP practice. This is part of the nationally recognised breast screening programme. Generally, women are invited for screening between their 50th and 53rd birthday. In some areas, however, women can be invited from the age of 47 as part of the trial extension of the programme (PHE 2015). There are also breast cancer assessment tools which help the clinician determine someone's risk of developing breast cancer (NICE 2011).

Risk factors for breast cancer

When considering risk factors, one needs to know the family history of breast cancer, particularly if the patient has a history of breast cancer in a first-degree relative. The BRCA1, BRCA2 and TP53 mutations carry very high risk, although environmental and lifestyle risk factors are also significant. The risk also increases with age. Other risk factors include:

- Never having borne a child or only having a first child after the age of 30
- Never having breast-fed
- Early menarche and late menopause
- Continuous combined HRT
- Radiation to chest
- Being overweight after the menopause
- High alcohol intake, which may increase risk in a dose-related manner.

Breast-feeding and physical activity may reduce risk. Breast augmentation is not generally associated with increased risk, though the type of implant used may be important.

Women are encouraged to be breast aware. The Department of Health (DH 2018) run a health campaign called 'Be breast aware' and their breast awareness five-point code is:
- Know what is normal for you
- Look and feel
- Know what changes to look for
- Report any changes without delay
- Attend for breast screening if aged 50 or over.

Breast care

Start by looking at your breasts in the mirror. Keep your shoulders straight and your arms on your hips. Examine the size, shape and colour of your breasts.

If you have any of the following changes, seek medical advice:
- Dimpling or orange-peel skin, puckering or bulging of the skin
- A nipple that has changed position or become inverted
- Redness, soreness, rash or swelling
- Any discharge from a nipple (such as a watery, milky or yellow fluid or blood discharge).

Then lie down and feel your breasts. Use your right hand to feel your left breast and then your left hand to feel your right breast. It is best to use a firm hand, with the first fingers of your hand flat and together. Using a circular motion (about the size of a ten-pence piece), check the whole area from top to bottom, side to side. It may be easiest to feel your breasts when the skin is wet and slippery.

(Adapted from Harding 2015)

Box 5.2: Breast care

Sociocultural concerns

There are also some sociocultural factors that prevent women and girls benefiting fully from health services (Bauer *et al.* 2000, Mosca *et al.* 2006, Scheppers *et al.* 2006).

These barriers can include:
- Unequal power relationships between men and women
- Social norms that decrease education and paid employment opportunities

- An exclusive focus on women's reproductive roles
- Potential or actual experience of physical, sexual and emotional violence.

(WHO 2018a).

There is a need for social welfare orientation and policy development to be conscious of these differences and support women's health (Raphael & Bryant 2004).

> ## Resources
>
> **Breast aware material:** https://www.breastcancercare.org.uk/information-support/have-i-got-breast-cancer/checking-your-breasts
>
> **DH Breast aware material:** https://assets.publishing.service.gov.uk/government/uploads/system/uploads/attachment_data/file/439602/breastaware.pdf
>
> **Find your local family planning service:** https://www.nhs.uk/Service-Search/Family%20planning/LocationSearch/1863
>
> **NHS contraception guide:** https://www.nhs.uk/conditions/contraception/
>
> **Sexual health guidelines from the British association for sexual health and HIV:** https://www.bashh.org/guidelines

Box 5.3: Resources

The following box provides the links to find out the answers for the reader activity 5.1.

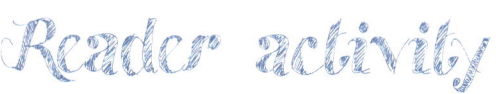 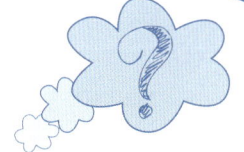

> You were asked to find out further information about the different methods of contraception.
> Here are some links so you can read about them:
> **https://www.nhs.uk/conditions/contraception/**
> **https://www.fpa.org.uk/**
> It would also be helpful to update your knowledge by reading the British Association for Sexual Health and HIV guidelines:
> **https://www.bashh.org/guidelines**

Box 5.4: Answers to reader activity – types of contraception

References

Bauer, H.M., Rodriguez, M.A., Quiroga, S.S. & Flores-Ortiz, Y.G. (2000). Barriers to health care for abused Latina and Asian immigrant women. *Journal of Health Care for the Poor and Underserved.* **11**(1), 33–44.

Cancer Research UK (2018). *Cancer Statistics for the UK.* https://www.cancerresearchuk.org/health-professional/cancer-statistics-for-the-uk (last accessed 5.2.2019).

DH (2018). Be breast aware, NHS cancer screening programme. https://assets.publishing.service.gov.uk/government/uploads/system/uploads/attachment_data/file/439602/breastaware.pdf (last accessed 5.1.2019).

Fehring, R.J., Schneider, M. & Raviele, K. (2006). Variability in the phases of the menstrual cycle. *Journal of Obstetric, Gynecologic & Neonatal Nursing.* **35**(3), 376–84.

Harding, M. (2015). Breast Lumps and Breast Examination. Patient Info. https://patient.info/doctor/Breast-Lumps-and-Breast-Examination (last accessed 5.1.2019).

Huisman, M., Kunst, A.E. & Mackenbach, J.P. (2005). Educational inequalities in smoking among men and women aged 16 years and older in 11 European countries. *Tobacco Control.* **14**(2), 106–13.

The Independent UK Panel on Breast Cancer Screening (IBSR) (2012). *The Benefits and Harms of Breast Cancer Screening: An Independent Review.* https://www.cancerresearchuk.org/sites/default/files/breast-screening-review-exec_0.pdf (last accessed 5.2.2019).

Kippley, J. & Kippley, S. (1996). *The art of family planning.* Couple to Couple League: UK.

Lawson, C.C., Whelan, E.A., Hibert, E.N.L., Spiegelman,D., Schernhammer, E.S. & Rich-Edwards, J.W. (2011). Rotating shift work and menstrual cycle characteristics. *Epidemiology* **22**(3), 305.

Mosca, L., Mochari, H., Christian, A., Berra, K., Taubert, K., Mills, T. & Simpson, S.L. (2006). National study of women's awareness, preventive action, and barriers to cardiovascular health. *Circulation.* **113**(4), 525–34.

Münster, K., Schmidt, L. & Helm, P. (1992). Length and variation in the menstrual cycle – a cross-sectional study from a Danish county. *BJOG: An International Journal of Obstetrics & Gynaecology.* **99**(5), 422–29.

NICE (2011). *Breast Cancer risk assessment tool.* https://www.cancer.gov/bcrisktool/Default.aspx (last accessed 5.1.2019).

NICE (2018). *Hormonal contraceptives.* https://bnf.nice.org.uk/treatment-summary/contraceptives-hormonal.html (last accessed 5.1.2019).

Public Health England (PHE) (2015). NHS breast screening (BSP) programme. https://www.gov.uk/topic/population-screening-programmes/breast (last accessed 5.1.2019).

Raphael, D. & Bryant, T. (2004). The welfare state as a determinant of women's health: support for women's quality of life in Canada and four comparison nations. *Health Policy.* **68**(1), 63–79.

Scheppers, E., van Dongen, E., Dekker, J., Geertzen, J. & Dekker, J. (2006). Potential barriers to the use of health services among ethnic minorities: a review. *Family Practice.* **23**(3), 1, 325–348. https://doi.org/10.1093/fampra/cmi113

Soriano, J.B., Maier, W.C., Egger, P., Visick, G., Thakrar, B., Sykes, J. & Pride, N.B. (2000). Recent trends in physician diagnosed COPD in women and men in the UK. *Thorax.* **55**(9), 789–94.

Wei, S., Schmidt, M.D., Dwyer, T., Norman, R.J. & Venn, A.J. (2009). Obesity and menstrual irregularity: associations with SHBG, testosterone, and insulin. *Obesity.* **17**(5), 1070–76.

Wilcox, A.J., Dunson, D. & Baird, D.D. (2000). The timing of the 'fertile window' in the menstrual cycle: day specific estimates from a prospective study. *British Medical Journal.* 321(7271), 1259–62.

Wild, S., Pierpoint, T., McKeigue, P. & Jacobs, H. (2000). Cardiovascular disease in women with polycystic ovary syndrome at long-term follow-up: a retrospective cohort study. *Clinical Endocrinology.* **52**(5), 595–600.

World Health Organization (WHO) (n.d.). Frequently asked questions. http://www.who.int/suggestions/faq/en/ (last accessed 5.1.2019).

World Health Organization (WHO) (2018a). Women's health. http://www.who.int/topics/womens_health/en/ (last accessed 5.1.2019).

World Health Organization (WHO) (2018b). Female genital mutilation. http://www.who.int/news-room/fact-sheets/detail/female-genital-mutilation (last accessed 5.1.2019).

Chapter 6

Men's health

Deborah Duncan

Introduction

Men have historically been poor at paying attention to their health. Compared to women, men are more likely to:

- Smoke and drink
- Make risky choices
- Fail to attend regular check-ups or to see their GP.

Certainly, men make less frequent use of medical services than women (Smith *et al.* 2006, Tudiver & Talbot 1999). They are also more likely to experience a cardiovascular event or to be affected by morbidity or mortality due to environmental factors (Smith *et al.* 2006). Men also experience more violence, unsafe sexual contact, smoking, alcohol and drug consumption; in addition, higher suicide rates contribute to premature death in more men than women (WHO 2018). The Global Burden of Disease study showed that, throughout the period from 1970 to 2010, women had a longer life expectancy than men (Rajaratnam *et al.* 2010).

Men's healthcare

Men's healthcare largely focuses on understanding how gender socialisation and masculine ideology affect men's health (Garfield *et al.* 2008). Generally, men are more likely than women to adopt beliefs and behaviours that increase their risks (Courtenay 2000). They are also less likely to engage in behaviours that will increase their life expectancy (Courtenay 2000).

Mahalik, Burns & Syzdek (2007) found that ideas about masculinity and the perceived normativeness of other men's health behaviours significantly affected their survey participants' own health behaviours. This influence was more significant than socio-demographic variables such as education, socio-economic group or income. In contrast, women's health behaviours were apparently unaffected by other participants' health behaviours. The key to supporting men's health appears to be education about self-examination and reducing risky behaviour.

Prostate conditions

The prostate is a small gland, the size of a walnut, found only in men in the pelvic area. It sits between the penis and the bladder and surrounds the urethra. The main function of the prostate gland is to produce a fluid that creates semen, once it is mixed with sperm. This fluid nourishes and transports sperm on their journey to meet the female ovum. The prostate also contracts and forces these fluids out during orgasm. The protein excreted by the prostate is called the prostate-specific antigen (PSA). Its role is to help semen retain its liquid state. It is also thought to be instrumental in dissolving cervical mucus and thus allowing sperm to progress to the uterus (Hellstrom 1999). A rise in the normal level of this protein in the blood is one of the first signs of prostate cancer.

Benign prostatic hyperplasia

Benign prostatic hyperplasia (BPH) is a non-cancerous increase in the size of the prostate. Symptoms are similar to those of prostate cancer, with frequent urination, trouble initiating flow, a weak stream, inability to urinate, or loss of bladder control. It can also lead to complications such as urinary tract infections, bladder stones and chronic kidney problems. The cause of BPH is unclear but risk factors include family history, obesity, type 2 diabetes and erectile dysfunction. It affects 50 per cent of men over the age of 50 (Kim *et al.* 2016).

The diagnosis of BPH is based on a history of lower urinary tract symptoms, a digital rectal exam, and the exclusion of other causes. An enlarged prostate gland on rectal examination is symmetrical and smooth. If the prostate gland feels asymmetrical, firm or nodular, then one needs to consider prostate cancer. Once diagnosed, patients can be prescribed medications such as pseudoephedrine, anticholinergics and calcium channel blockers. It is a case of discovering which medication helps, as some can cause the symptoms to worsen.

Prostate cancer

If a patient has a raised specific antigen (PSA) level, positive digital rectal examination (DRE) findings and risk factors (including increasing age and black Afro-Caribbean family origin), they should be offered an examination of the prostate. This is not offered on the serum PSA level alone (NICE 2014).

There are usually no symptoms during the early stages of prostate cancer. Common symptoms include:

- Frequent urges to urinate during the day and night
- Difficulty in commencing and maintaining urinary flow
- Presence of blood in the urine
- Pain on micturition and occasionally on ejaculation
- Problems in achieving or maintaining an erection.

Table 6.1: Risk stratification for men with localised prostate cancer
(Adapted from NICE 2014)

Level of risk	PSA		Gleason score		Clinical stage
Low risk	<10 ng/ml	and	≤6	and	T1–T2a
Intermediate risk	10–20 ng/ml	or	7	or	T2b
High risk*	>20 ng/ml	or	8–10	or	≥T2c

*High-risk localised prostate cancer is also included in the definition of locally advanced prostate cancer.

In more advanced cases, men can experience bone pain (often in the spine, femur, pelvis or ribs), bone fractures and then compression on the spinal column. This can lead to urinary incontinence, faecal incontinence and leg weakness.

There are various treatment options, depending on the requirements of individual cases. Initially, in early prostate cancer it is a case of watchful waiting or monitoring as the PSA blood levels are regularly checked. This is because the risk of treatment side effects outweighs the risk of watching and waiting.

In the early stages, patients may receive radiation therapy combined with hormone therapy for up to six months.

Radical prostatectomy or radical radiotherapy is offered to men with an intermediate risk of localised prostate cancer. It is also offered to men with high-risk localised prostate cancer when there is a realistic prospect of long-term disease control. During a radical prostatectomy the prostate is surgically removed. Brachytherapy can also be performed. In this procedure, radioactive seeds are implanted into the prostate to deliver targeted radiation treatment.

There is also conformal radiation therapy, in which the radiation beams are shaped so that the region where they overlap is as close to the same shape as the organ or region that requires treatment or intensity modulated radiation therapy (in which variable-intensity beams are used).

There are adverse effects associated with the radical treatment options. Patients should be referred for specialist support. These conditions include:

- Sexual dysfunction
- Urinary incontinence
- Radiation-induced enteropathy.

As a GPN, you may meet patients who are receiving intermittent long-term androgen deprivation therapy. They have their specific antigen (PSA) tested every three months and receive injectable androgen deprivation therapy if their PSA is 10 ng/ml or above, or if there is symptomatic progression (NICE 2014). The most common form of this injectable hormone therapy or implant is Goserelin acetate (brand name Zoladex), which suppresses the hormone testosterone.

> ## Reader activity
>
> Look at the guidelines for hormonal injectable therapy Goserelin acetate (Zoladex). Find out what you commonly give in your practice. You will not be able to administer this until you have the appropriate training. Review the instructions with your mentor.

Box 6.1: Reader activity – Goserelin acetate

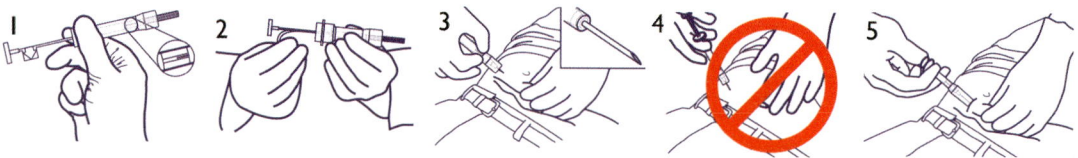

Figure 6.1: Goserelin acetate (Zoladex) being administered

Scrotal swellings

The common or important causes of scrotal swelling include:

- Testicular cancer
- Squamous cell carcinoma of the scrotum
- Testicular torsion (torsion of spermatic cord)
- Torsion of a testicular or epididymal appendage
- Epididymo-orchitis
- Epididymal cyst, or spermatocele
- Varicocele
- Hydrocele
- Haematocele.

Diagnosis is made according to symptoms, including:

- Presence of pain, its duration, and severity
- Speed of onset of pain and swelling
- Previous episodes of severe, self-limiting pain and swelling
- Associated symptoms, including symptoms of a lower urinary tract infection, or urethral discharge, parotid swelling, or nausea or vomiting
- History of trauma.

There should be a low threshold for suspecting testicular torsion in a male under the age of 30 presenting with acute, painful scrotal swelling (NICE 2017b).

If testicular torsion, or torsion of an appendage of the testis or epididymis, is suspected, the person should be admitted to hospital immediately (to urology or paediatric surgery). They also need to be referred if there is any diagnostic uncertainty.

Testicular cancer

If a man has suspected testicular cancer, clinicians should fulfil the suspected cancer pathway referral (for an appointment within two weeks), particularly if they have a non-painful enlargement or change in shape or texture of the testis (NICE 2017a). They should be referred for a direct access ultrasound scan for testicular cancer.

The symptoms caused by testicular cancer symptoms are the same as other conditions that affect the testicles. Men are taught to watch out for:

- A lump or swelling in the testicle
- Any unusual difference between one testicle and the other

- A 'heavy' feeling scrotum
- Discomfort or pain in a testicle or the scrotum
- Testicular cancer is not usually painful but the first symptom for some men is a sharp pain in the testicle or scrotum
- If the cancer has spread to the lymph glands, patients may experience backache or a dull ache in the abdomen.

Diagnosing testicular cancer

The clinician will need to assess the patient. They will need to determine whether there is any tenderness. Then they will need to inspect, auscultate and palpate like any other examination. They are looking for:

- The position of the swelling in relation to the testis
- The testicular lie
- Size of the testis
- Consistency of the swelling
- Lymphadenopathy or an abdominal mass
- Cremasteric reflex
- Features of inguinal hernia (both lying and standing)
- Skin changes.

Transillumination

Transillumination is a simple non-invasive test. A strong light is shone through the testicle. If the light shows through it, the lump is a harmless, fluid-filled cyst called a hydrocele. If the light can't shine through, it is more likely to be cancer, which is a solid mass.

Prehn's sign

Prehn's sign involves physically lifting the testicles and assessing for pain. A negative Prehn's sign means that pain is not relieved by lifting the affected testicle. This points towards testicular torsion, which is a surgical emergency. A positive Prehn's sign means that pain is relieved by lifting the affected testicle, and this indicates epididymitis.

As in women's health, the main aid to prevention is self-examination. Men should be taught to carry out self-examination for testicular cancer at a young age. It is best performed after a warm bath or shower as heat relaxes the scrotum, therefore making it easier to feel or see anything abnormal.

Self-examination for testicular cancer

- Stand in front of a mirror.
- Check for any swelling on the scrotal skin. Free-floating lumps in the scrotum that are not attached to a testicle are not testicular cancer.
- Examine each testicle with both hands. Place the index and middle fingers under the testicle with the thumbs placed on top. Roll the testicle gently between the thumbs and fingers. This should not be painful. One testicle may seem slightly larger than the other – this is normal.
- Find the epididymis, the soft, tube-like structure behind the testicle that collects and carries sperm.
- If you have any concerns, check with a medical practitioner!

Box 6.2: Self-examination of the testes (Adapted from BAUS 2017).

Box 6.2 (above) explains how to perform a self-examination of the testes. It is recommended that pubescent boys should be taught to self-examine (BAUS 2017). The following figure illustrates this procedure.

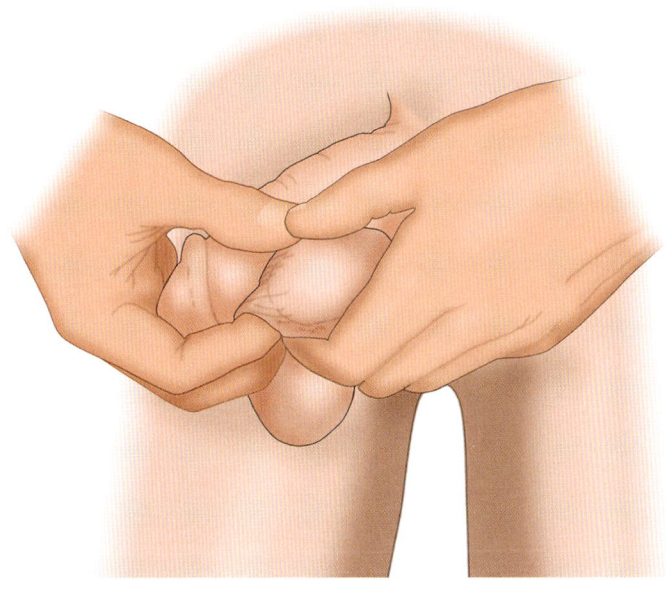

Figure 6.2: Self-examination of the testes.

> **Resources**
> **Testicular cancer:**
> https://www.cancerresearchuk.org/about-cancer/testicular-cancer/symptoms
> **Macmillan self-examination for testicular cancer:** https://www.macmillan.org.uk/information-and-support/testicular-cancer/understanding-cancer/testicular-self-examination.html
> **BAUS self-examination:** https://www.baus.org.uk/_userfiles/pages/files/Patients/Leaflets/Testicular%20self%20examination.pdf

Box 6.3: Resources

Erectile dysfunction (ED)

We often presume that this topic is one our patients are unwilling to discuss; yet it has been found that health professionals do not discuss sexually related issues in consultations as often as patients would like (Gott *et al.* 2004). Primary care is the preferred place to seek treatment for sexual health concerns so, as general practice nurses, we need to be able to initiate such discussions. In fact the Royal College of Nursing states that sexual health is part of the holistic care of patients and clients (RCN 2001).

An example of this reticence often occurs when reviewing patients with type 2 diabetes. We know that erectile dysfunction is a complication of diabetes, yet we do not always ask patients if they have problems in that area. In Almigbal & Schattner's 2018 study, their male patients with type 2 diabetes were not asked about ED within the last year of attendance even though most were willing to discuss it with their physicians.

The Clinical Knowledge Summaries (NICE 2017c) offer the following guidance for men attending with ED. They suggest identifying and treating any modifiable risk factors which include lifestyle or drug-related factors for ED. They also suggest ensuring that any underlying conditions, such as diabetes or hypertension, are well controlled. The guidance for referral is in Box 6.4.

> ## Referral pathway for erectile dysfunction
> 1. Admit to hospital if there is priapism (persistent erection)
> 2. Arrange referral:
> - To urology – for young men who have always had difficulty in obtaining or maintaining an erection; for men with a history of trauma (for example to the genital area, pelvis or spine); if an abnormality of the penis or testicles is found on examination

- To endocrinology – for men who have hypogonadism (where there is abnormal testosterone, follicle-stimulating hormone, luteinizing hormone, or prolactin levels)
- To cardiology – for men who have severe/unstable cardiovascular disease (CVD) that would make sexual activity unsafe or contraindicated
- For the use of phosphodiesterase-5 (PDE-5) inhibitor use (such as high-risk arrhythmias, unstable or refractory angina, or recent myocardial infarction)
- To mental health services – for men with a psychogenic underlying cause of erectile dysfunction and those with severe mental distress.

Box 6.4: Erectile dysfunction pathway
(Adapted from NICE 2017c)

Summary

The key to supporting men's health appears to be education about self-examination and reducing risky behaviour. GPNs also need to be more confident in initiating conversations about sexual health and issues pertinent to men's health such as erectile dysfunction.

References

Almigbal, T. & Schattner, P. (21018). The willingness of Saudi men with type 2 diabetes to discuss erectile dysfunction with their physicians and the factors that influence this. *PLOS.* https://doi.org/10.1371/journal.pone.0201105 (last accessed 8.1.2019).

British Association of Urological Surgeons (BAUS) (2017). *Testicular Self-examination.* https://www.baus.org.uk/_userfiles/pages/files/Patients/Leaflets/Testicular%20self%20examination.pdf (last accessed 8.1.2019).

Courtenay, W.H. (2000). Constructions of masculinity and their influence on men's well-being: a theory of gender and health. *Social Science and Medicine.* **50**(10), 1385–1401.

Garfield, C.F., Isacco, A. & Rogers, T.E. (2008). A review of men's health and masculinity. *American Journal of Lifestyle Medicine.* **2**(6), 474–87.

Gott, M., Galena, E., Hinchliff, S. & Elford, H. (2004). 'Opening a can of worms': GP and practice nurse barriers to talking about sexual health in primary care. *Family Practice.* **21**(5), 528–36.

Hellstrom, W.J.G. (ed.) (1999). Chapter 8: What is the prostate and what is its function? *American Society of Andrology Handbook.* San Francisco: American Society of Andrology. ISBN 1-891276-02-6.

Kim, E.H., Larson, J.A. & Andriole, G.L. (2016). Management of Benign Prostatic Hyperplasia. *Annual Review of Medicine (Review).* **67**, 137–51. doi:10.1146/annurev-med-063014-123902. PMID 26331999

Mahalik, J.R., Burns, S.M. & Syzdek, M. (2007). Masculinity and perceived normative health behaviors as predictors of men's health behaviors. *Social Science and Medicine.* **64**(11), 2201–2209.

NICE (2014). Prostate cancer: diagnosis and management. Clinical guideline [CG175]. https://www.nice.org.uk/guidance/cg175/chapter/1-Recommendations#assessment-2 (last accessed 8.1.2019).

NICE (2017a). Suspected cancer: recognition and referral. NICE guideline [NG12]. https://www.nice.org.uk/guidance/ng12/chapter/terms-used-in-this-guideline#terms-used-in-this-guideline (last accessed 8.1.2019).

NICE (2017b). Scrotal swellings. Clinical Knowledge Summaries. https://cks.nice.org.uk/scrotal-swellings#!topicsummary (last accessed 8.1.2019).

NICE (2017c). Erectile dysfunction. https://cks.nice.org.uk/erectile-dysfunction#!scenario (last accessed 8.1.2019).

Rajaratnam, J.K., Marcus, J.R., Levin-Rector, A., Chalupka, A.N., Wang, H., et al. (2010). Worldwide mortality in men and women aged 15–59 years from 1970 to 2010: a systematic analysis. *The Lancet.* **375**(9727), 1704–20.

Royal College of Nursing (RCN) (2001). *Royal College of Nursing Sexual Health Strategy: Guidance for Nursing Staff.* London: RCN.

Smith, J., Braunack-Mayer, A. & Wittert, G. (2006). What do we know about men's help-seeking and health service use? *The Medical Journal of Australia.* **184**(2), 81–83.

Tudiver, F. & Talbot, Y. (1999). Why don't men seek help? Family physician's perspectives on help seeking behaviour in men. *Journal of Family Practice.* **48**, 47–52.

World Health Organization (WHO) (2018). Men's health. http://www.euro.who.int/en/health-topics/health-determinants/gender/activities/mens-health (last accessed 8.1.2019).

Chapter 7

Immunisation

Jacqueline Johnstone

Introduction

Immunisation, also referred to as vaccination, is the greatest single health promotion and health sector intervention (WHO 2005). Diseases considered to be common in childhood a few generations ago, such as mumps, polio, pertussis and measles, are now (thankfully) quite rare in the UK. Indeed, many young mothers may not have even heard of some of the previously named infectious diseases. Diseases like smallpox have been eradicated and outbreaks of others (such as polio) are rare in developed countries with robust immunisation programmes, as are adverse outcomes.

Nevertheless, outbreaks of these diseases often make news headlines; and recent news reports have focused on the increased occurrence of measles. For instance, the 2018 measles outbreak in England was linked to a Europe-wide outbreak and Duncan Selbie, Chief Executive of Public Health England, said (PHE 2018):

> Until measles is eliminated from all WHO regions, cross-border transmission of cases is likely to occur when unvaccinated individuals travel to countries where measles is circulating, become infected and travel back to their home country – thus importing the measles virus.

This chapter will discuss immunity and mainly focus on the vaccination schedule for infants aged up to 12 months. Relevant details of the associated diseases will also be summarised; and public perception and controversies regarding immunisation as a public health measure will be explored.

Controversy and public perception

It is perhaps an inevitable consequence of the success of any immunisation programme, with the aim of eradicating a particular disease, that subsequent generations have no concept of the disease and its dangers to the health and long-term wellbeing of individuals. This, along with other influencing factors, may explain the relaxation of uptake by parents. Unfounded scare stories about the side effects of vaccinations, and the perception that vaccinations are unsafe, with more side effects than other types of medications and a greater risk of complications than contracting the infectious disease, appear to be common. On any given social media platform, a barrage of 'expert testimonials' will be given regarding vaccinations and their supposed dangers.

In the UK, an infamous example of 'scaremongering' came from a source commonly referred to as 'The Wakefield Study' (Wakefield *et al.* 1998). This article was published in a medical journal and was then picked up by the media, under headlines such as 'MMR causes autism – direct link'. Public health response to this misguided media coverage was swift, with analysis of the deficiencies of the (subsequently retracted) study, and refuted research. However, a large section of the public elected to believe the media rather than the public health information and uptake of the MMR vaccination subsequently declined. The retraction of the article, and Wakefield's removal from the Medical Register, did not achieve the same level of media attention and Wakefield is still frequently quoted by his supporters.

Indeed, some 'anti-imms' campaigners may feel that Wakefield has been vilified for speaking out or that he was also a victim of media misrepresentation. A statement from the retracted article could be used to support this view: 'We did not prove an association between measles, mumps, and rubella vaccine and the syndrome described' (Wakefield *et al.* 1998, p 641). However, this statement could refer to links implying that MMR immunisation causes Crohn's disease only.

Whilst the media and wider social media may bear some responsibility, so too perhaps does the terminology used by health sectors, which is subsequently, potentially, picked up and used incorrectly by the media. For instance, in 2017 the World Health Organization declared that the United Kingdom had successfully 'eliminated measles' (GOV.UK 2018a).

In GOV.UK (2018a) Selbie *et al.* continue to explain that elimination does not mean that measles has disappeared. Measles continues to be endemic in many countries and can therefore continue to be imported into the UK. If the MMR vaccination uptake is below 95 per cent, herd immunity is not achieved, and UK outbreaks will continue.

Table 7.1 shows the uptake of scheduled vaccinations in the UK, and Table 7.2 shows the uptake specifically of the MMR vaccination. Whilst there has been a general

Immunisation

rise in vaccination uptake, this is inconsistent. Although Northern Ireland, Scotland and Wales continue to achieve the 95 per cent herd immunity target, England only achieves this for some of the scheduled vaccinations and has never in the last 8 years achieved 95 per cent herd immunity, with the uptake for MMR being particularly low. This country variation in uptake is interesting, given that these countries broadly share the same media outlets and National Health Service, even though there may be some local news outlets and variations in health services.

Table 7.1: NHS childhood vaccine coverage statistics *(NHS 2018a)*

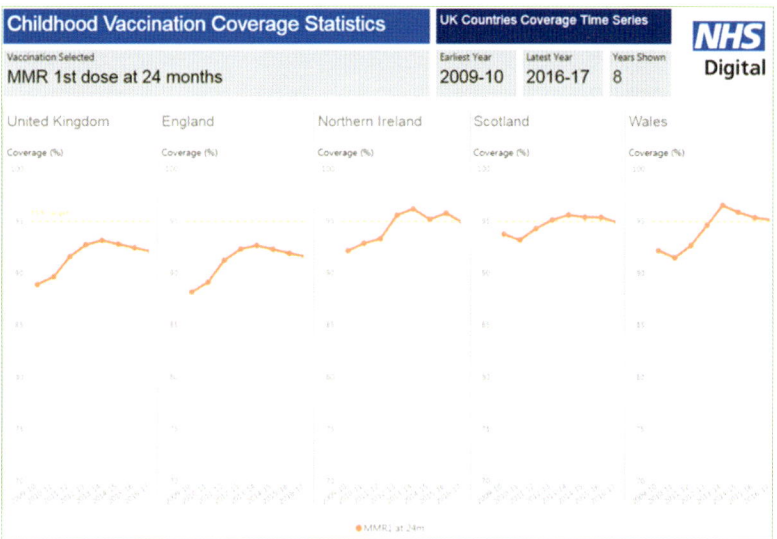

Table 7.2: Childhood MMR vaccine coverage *(NHS 2018a)*

Vaccination and the greater good?

The aim of a vaccination programme is to eradicate, eliminate and contain any disease outbreak for the population. Perhaps one of the factors in a parent's refusal to immunise their child is the belief that the vaccine has 'no benefit' to that child but could in fact cause harm. This contrasts with other types of medication, which are prescribed and administered for immediate benefit, to treat or prophylactically reduce an immediate risk from a specific condition. Immunisations are given to the 'well child', in the hope that herd immunity will eradicate the spread of the disease. Cane (1999), in Jackson (2016), uses the example of pertussis as a disease and the vaccinations schedule which exemplifies the 'free-rider' problem and herd immunity, in that the pertussis vaccination is given to the child at a time when their contracting the disease would be unlikely to be fatal. The individual is therefore being vaccinated to reduce the risk they could pose to others. This leads to an argument about children being used to protect others, before they have the ability to understand the concept and consequences. Also, parents may feel that the risk of having their children vaccinated is greater than the risk of them actually contracting the disease.

Reader activity

Case study: Albie is 7 weeks old and he is currently in temporary foster care as his mother is complying with her current methadone drug withdrawal programme. Albie has two older siblings who are also in temporary foster care. During a pre-immunisation discussion, Ruby, Albie's mother, states that she does not consent to Albie having his immunisations.

Consider and reflect:
- What information would you want from Ruby?
- What information would you give Ruby?
- What further actions would you consider?
- Who would you discuss this issue with, and what input would you expect them to have?
- How do you feel about this situation?
- Does your area of practice have guidelines for such circumstances?

Box 7.1: Reader activity – case study

Jackson (2016) discusses the ethics of vaccinations and the special state compensation for individuals who are permanently adversely affected because of general vaccination schedules. However, there have been very few successful claims and the legal system appears to take the view that immunisations are beneficial to the individual and directly protect them. In Re SL (Wilson 2017) the court decided that the child had a right to have their health protected by way of vaccination.

Immunity

Immunity is the body's ability to protect itself from infectious diseases and harmful pathogens. Immunity can be innate or acquired. Innate immunity is non-specific and non-adaptive. This involves the body's 'warriors' (macrophages and neutrophils) which have a set procedure (phagocytosis) for recognising and dealing with certain kinds of infection. No previous exposure to, or memory of, the specific disease is required. Innate immunity can be present from birth and includes physical barriers (such as intact skin) and chemical barriers (for example, digestive enzymes). This innate immunity is often referred to as the 'first line of defence'.

Acquired or adaptive immunity is the process in which antibodies are formed in response to a specific disease or germ. This may be either passive or active. Passive immunity occurs when antibodies are directly transferred into the non-immune individual. This occurs with maternal to foetal antibody transfer or when immunoglobulins are administered to specific patients. Active immunity requires time and can occur when the individual is exposed to the disease or when a vaccination is administered. This aspect of immunity requires time for the body to recognise and adapt to the infection; once the disease has been 'learned', the production of antibodies ensures that any future exposure triggers a rapid and effective immune response.

Vaccinations stimulate the immune response and the production of antibodies. This gives the individual protection without them having to experience the dangers of a real infection. However, the 'memory' produced by immunisations may not last as long as that generated by exposure to the disease. As detailed in Table 7.3 below, vaccinations can be live or inactive and both types may require booster injections. Despite individuals receiving a full immunisation schedule and booster updates, a small percentage of fully vaccinated individuals will still become infected by a 'vaccinated' disease. This vaccine failure can be primary or secondary. Primary failure is when there is no initial immune response to the vaccine. Secondary failure occurs when the initial immune response diminishes over time and the individual goes on to contract the disease (PHE 2018).

General Practice Nursing

Reader activity

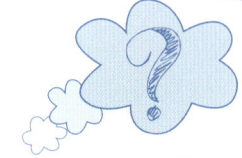

Take time to consider and reflect on the following questions. Discuss them with your mentor.

How would you respond to a parent who tells you:
- Immunisations do not work?
- Immunisations put their child at risk for no benefit?
- It is better for the child to contract the disease?
- It isn't safe to have so many medicines at once?
- Their baby is unwell and therefore cannot be vaccinated?

What other questions do you think parents may have, concerning vaccinations and the schedule?

Box 7.2: Reader activity – questions

Diseases

As previously discussed, immunisations are not perfect, and controversies and ethical debates continue. It appears to be a battle to achieve and maintain the 95 per cent herd immunity target, as detailed in Tables 7.1 and 7.2. It is therefore worth reviewing the diseases that the immunisation schedule aims to eradicate, contain and eliminate. Table 7.3 provides key information about these diseases, their signs and symptoms and complications.

Table 7.3: Diseases that we immunise against

Disease	Prevalence	Spread	Complications	Signs and symptoms
Diphtheria	Rare in the UK due to vaccination programmes. Cases still prevalent throughout the world	Air — coughs/sneezes. Close contact with, or sharing items with, an infected person	Highly contagious and can be fatal. Can be local or systemic. Local — formation of membrane impacting on the nose, pharynx and larynx. Systemic — cardiac and neurological disturbances	2–5 days post infection: • Sore throat and a thick grey-white coating at back of throat • Swollen neck glands • Pyrexia — 38°C or above • Nausea • Headache • Breathing and swallowing difficulties Possibly — • Ulcers

Tetanus	Rare in the UK due to vaccination programmes	Tetanus bacteria from soil and manure getting into a wound Contaminated drug injections	Severe Untreated or expose encountered by those not fully vaccinated Immunoglobulin therapy Intensive care admission	4 to 21 days post infection: • Muscle stiffness and spasm • Breathing and swallowing difficulties • Pyrexia • Tachycardia
Pertussis (Whooping Cough)	Endemic Epidemics every few years due to falling vaccination uptakes Secondary failure due to vaccine's lifespan Pregnant women may be offered a booster vaccination	Bordetella pertussis — Air (coughs/sneezes)	Highly contagious and can be fatal Dehydration Pneumonia Seizures Renal and brain damage	Initially cold-like symptoms Intense coughing bouts start about a week later: • Paroxysmal cough followed by inspiratory whoop and vomit • Paroxysmal cough followed by apnoea in infants • Epistaxis
Polio	Almost eradicated worldwide	Air — coughs/sneezes Contact — faeces of someone infected with Poliovirus Or contaminated food and water Rare — however, noted cases of infection due to live vaccination (oral vaccination)	Permanent paralysis Joint contractures Muscle atrophy Post-Polio syndrome	Asymptomatic — majority Minority of infected individual may develop flu-like symptoms with nausea 3—21 days post infection, usually lasting a week < 1 per cent of those infected • Paralytic poliomyelitis
Hib	Rare	Haemophilus influenzae type b (Hib) bacterium Air — coughs/sneezes	Serious • Meningitis • Septicaemia • Pneumonia • Pericarditis • Epiglottitis • Septic arthritis • Cellulitis • Osteomyelitis	Healthy individuals can be asymptomatic to Haemophilus influenzae type b (Hib) bacterium in the airway Symptoms specific to complication developed by young, vulnerable and unimmunised individuals
Hepatitis B	Low in the UK	Hepatitis B virus Contact with body fluids of contaminated individual	Protects against: • Cirrhosis • Liver cancer	Symptoms specific to complication developed by young, vulnerable and unimmunised individuals
Meningitis C	Low in the UK	Bacterial or viral air — coughs/sneezes Close contact with, or sharing items with, an infected person	Bacterial — serious • Septicaemia • Neurological damage	• Pyrexia • Nausea • Rash • Stiff neck • Photosensitivity • Seizure • Drowsiness or unresponsiveness

Pneumococcal infection	Prior to the immunisation being introduced into the vaccination schedule >500 cases of infected children under the age of 2 years per annum in England	Streptococcus pneumoniae bacterium	Serious and can be fatal • Pneumonia • Septicaemia • Meningitis	Symptoms specific to complication developed
Rotavirus	Prevalent prior to the immunisation being introduced into the vaccination schedule	Highly infectious	Rare Dehydration	• Diarrhoea • Nausea • Stomach cramps • Pyrexia • Dehydration
Measles	Eradicated in UK; however, notifications of disease in the UK	Air – coughs/sneezes Contact with surfaces with settled droplets and then touching mouth or nose Virus survives on surfaces for hours	Serious and can be fatal • Pneumonia • Encephalitis	• Nausea • Cold-like symptoms, • Photosensitivity • Conjunctivitis • Koplik spots • Maculopapular rash • Pyrexia
Mumps	Prevalent prior to the immunisation being introduced into the vaccination schedule	Contagious viral infection Air – Coughs/sneezes Contact with surfaces with settled droplets and then touching mouth or nose	Rare • Swollen testicles or ovaries • Viral meningitis • Pancreatitis pneumonia • Encephalitis • Hearing loss	Develop 14–25 days post infection: • Parotid gland swelling • Headache • Joint pain • Nausea • Abdominal pain • Lethargy • Pyrexia • Loss of appetite
Rubella (German measles)	Prevalent prior to the immunisation being introduced into the vaccination schedule	Togavirus Air – coughs/sneezes Contact with surfaces with settled droplets and then touching mouth or nose	Rare Serious risk to foetus if virus contracted by pregnant female	Develop 14–21 days post infection: • Maculopapular rash • Lymphadenopathy • Cold-like symptoms • Joint pain • Abdominal pain • Lethargy • Pyrexia • Loss of appetite

National immunisation programme

Differences in immunisation schedules exist from country to country. The schedule may be patient-specific or condition-specific – for example, pre-term infants should have their scheduled immunisations based on their actual date of birth, rather than their due date or their corrected age (NICE 2019). Schedules may also alter with the introduction of new vaccines or research findings. For instance, a relatively recent addition to the schedule is the rotavirus vaccine. The latest editions of the Green Book and the BNFc should always be consulted. Practitioners with internet access may find it useful to access the Department of Health Immunisation Schedule pages (GOV.UK 2018b).

There is a useful tool for parents, a vaccination planner (see Figure 7.1). The infant's immunisation history may also be available in the patient's hand-held 'red book', although this is not a UK-wide resource. In the absence of a complete vaccination schedule, as well as a patient assessment, it is vital to take a thorough patient history. Where the routine childhood vaccination programme has not been completed, any remaining doses should be given (BNFc 2017–18). An algorithm detailing the process for patients with an incomplete or unknown vaccination status is available from Public Health England (PHE 2017).

Guidance on immunisation protocols for children who come into the UK can be found on the Department of Health website and information on specific country's immunisation schedules can be found on the World Health Organization website (WHO 2018). The current UK schedule for infants up to the age of one year is detailed in Table 7.4 and Table 7.5 details the process for patient-specific immunisations.

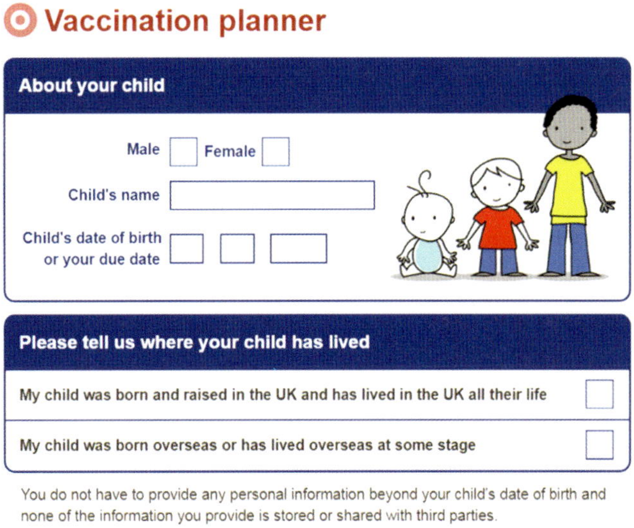
Vaccination planner

About your child

Male ☐ Female ☐

Child's name

Child's date of birth or your due date

Please tell us where your child has lived

My child was born and raised in the UK and has lived in the UK all their life ☐

My child was born overseas or has lived overseas at some stage ☐

You do not have to provide any personal information beyond your child's date of birth and none of the information you provide is stored or shared with third parties.

Figure 7.1: Department of Health Vaccination Planner (NHS 2016)

Table 7.4: Immunisation schedule for infants aged up to one year

Age immunisation due	Vaccination to be administered	Disease immunity against	Mode and site of administration
2 months old	DtaP/IPV/Hib/HepB	Diphtheria, tetanus, pertussis (whooping cough), polio, Haemophilus influenza type b (Hib) and hepatitis B	Intramuscular injection Thigh – anterolateral
	Pneumococcal conjugate vaccine (PCV)	Pneumococcal (13 serotypes)	Intramuscular injection Thigh – anterolateral
	MenB	Meningococcal group B (MenB)	Intramuscular injection LEFT thigh – anterolateral
	Rotavirus	Rotavirus gastroenteritis	Orally – to be taken by mouth
3 months old	DtaP/IPV/Hib/HepB	Diphtheria, tetanus, pertussis (whooping cough), polio, Haemophilus influenza type b (Hib) and hepatitis B	Intramuscular injection Thigh – anterolateral
	Rotavirus	Rotavirus gastroenteritis	Orally – to be taken by mouth
4 months old	DtaP/IPV/Hib/HepB	Diphtheria, tetanus, pertussis (whooping cough), polio, Haemophilus influenza type b (Hib) and hepatitis B	Intramuscular injection Thigh – anterolateral
	PCV	Pneumococcal (13 serotypes)	Intramuscular injection Thigh – anterolateral
	MenB	MenB	Intramuscular injection LEFT thigh – anterolateral
12–13 months old	Hib/MenC	Hib and MenC	Intramuscular injection upper arm or thigh
	PCV	Pneumococcal (13 serotypes)	Intramuscular injection upper arm or thigh
	MMR	Measles, mumps and Rubella (German measles)	Intramuscular injection upper arm or thigh
	MenB Booster	MenB	Intramuscular injection LEFT thigh – anterolateral
Denotes live vaccine			

(Adapted from GOV.UK 2018 and BNFc 2017–18)

Table 7.5: Selective immunisation schedule for infants

Immunisation Schedule			
Babies born to hepatitis B infected mothers	At birth, four weeks and 12 months old [1,2]	Hepatitis B	Hepatitis B (Engerix B/HBvaxPRO)
Infants in areas of the country with TB incidence >=40/100,000	At birth	Tuberculosis	BCG
Infants with a parent or grandparent born in a high incidence country [3]	At birth	Tuberculosis	BCG
1. Take blood for HBsAG at 12 months to exclude infection 2. In addition hexavalent vaccine (infanrix hexa) is given at 8, 12 and 16 weeks 3. Where the annual incidence of TBn is >=40/100,000 — see www.gov.uk/government/publications/tuberculosis-tb-by-country-rates-per-100000-people			

(Adapted from GOV.UK 2018)

Immunisation administration

Healthcare professionals involved in discussions, education, consent-taking, preparation and administration of immunisations must receive specific training in vaccinations and anaphylaxis. As with any other aspect of professional practice, it is the practitioner's responsibility to keep up to date.

This involves utilising online resources to ensure that vaccination practice and care are current, including:

- Preparation and storage of vaccinations
- Cold chain
- Administration – before, during and after
- Parental information.

Contraindications and special considerations

Although vaccinations are safe, there are some contraindications and special considerations associated with each vaccination (as with any drug). In complex contraindicated patients, a senior paediatrician or immunisation lead should be consulted prior to a decision being made on withholding the vaccination. In cases of a previous episode of anaphylaxis following a vaccination, the individual should not receive that specific immunisation again. However, other vaccinations can be given (Salisbury *et al.* 2017).

Vaccination side effects

All medications have side effects and immunisations are no different. Parents must be informed of these side effects and the appropriate management strategies.

Table 7.6: Management of potential side effects

Side effect	Management
• Swelling, redness or a small lump at the injection site • Redness	• Can last 2–3 days – no treatment required
• Pyrexia	• Check temperature with a thermometer If there is a high temperature: • Keep clothing and bedding to a minimum • Breastfeed or give cool fluids • Sponge baby and nurse near a fan • Give paracetamol following the MenB vaccination

Summary

This chapter has discussed the diseases and related vaccination schedules for infants from birth until 12 months in the UK. The controversies surrounding vaccinations and ethical principles have been considered and there have been opportunities to reflect on current knowledge and thoughts surrounding vaccinations. Further details of vaccinations can be found in the Green Book resource. The normal schedule is regularly updated – please ensure that you check the most recent one (see Box 7.3 below).

Resources

The Green Book: https://www.gov.uk/government/collections/immunisation-against-infectious-disease-the-green-book (last accessed 16.1.2019)

Normal schedule: https://assets.publishing.service.gov.uk/government/uploads/system/uploads/attachment_data/file/699392/Complete_immunisation_schedule_april2018.pdf (last accessed 16.1.2019)

Box 7.3: Resources

References

Australian Immunisation Handbook. http://immunise.health.gov.au/internet/immunise/publishing.nsf/Content/7B28E87511E08905CA257D4D001DB1F8/$File/Aus-Imm-Handbook.pdf (last accessed 16.1.2019).

GOV.UK (2018a). https://publichealthmatters.blog.gov.uk/2018/01/22/measles-has-been-eliminated-in-the-uk-so-why-do-we-still-see-cases-and-outbreaks/ (last accessed 16.1.2019)

GOV.UK (2018b). https://www.gov.uk/government/publications/the-complete-routine-immunisation-schedule (last accessed 16.1.2019).

Jackson, E. (2016). *Medical Law.* 4th edn. Oxford: Oxford University Press.

Lissauer, T. & Carroll, W. (2017). *Illustrated Textbook of Paediatrics.* 5th edn. Elsevier.

NHS (2016). https://www.nhs.uk/Tools/Pages/NHSvaccinationplanner.aspx (last accessed 15.1.2019).

NHS (2018a). *Childhood Vaccination Coverage Statistics, England, 2016–17* NHS Digital https://digital.nhs.uk/data-and-information/publications/statistical/childhood-vaccination-coverage-statistics/childhood-vaccination-coverage-statistics-england-2016-17 (last accessed 16.1.2019)

NHS (2018b). https://assets.publishing.service.gov.uk/government/uploads/system/uploads/attachment_data/file/699392/Complete_immunisation_schedule_april2018.pdf (last accessed 16.1.2019)

NICE (2019). *BNF for Children.* https://bnfc.nice.org.uk/ (last accessed 16.1.2019).

Public Health England (PHE) (2017). https://assets.publishing.service.gov.uk/government/uploads/system/uploads/attachment_data/file/658744/Algorithm_of_individuals_with_uncertain_or_incomplete_vaccine_status.pdf (last accessed 16.1.2019).

Public Health England (PHE) (2018). *Measles: why it is necessary to eliminate the disease in Europe Public Health England and the Italian National Health Institute stress the need to eradicate the disease from all European countries. 19 July 2018.* https://www.gov.uk/government/news/measles-why-it-is-necessary-to-eliminate-the-disease-in-europe (last accessed 16.1.2019).

Wilson, T. (2017). *Re SL (Permission to Vaccinate) (2017).* EWHC 125 (Fam) https://www.familylawweek.co.uk/site.aspx?i=ed175768 (last accessed 23/01/2019).

Wakefield, A.J., Murch, S.H., *et al.* (1998). Ileal-lymphoid-nodular hyperplasia, non-specific colitis, and pervasive developmental disorder in children. *Lancet.* **351**(9103), 637–41.

World Health Organization (WHO) (2005). http://www.who.int/topics/immunization/en/ (last accessed 16.1.2019).

World Health Organization (WHO) (2018). http://apps.who.int/immunization_monitoring/globalsummary/ (last accessed 16.1.2019).

Chapter 8

Travel health

Deborah Duncan

Introduction

The GPN is often the first person a potential traveller will see to discuss travel vaccinations (Zuckerman 2002). Not all surgeries offer this service but the GPN needs to know how to give general advice and where to refer the client. What services are available in your local area? There are some general points to consider.

General information

The patient should be reassured that the overall risk of contracting infectious diseases when travelling abroad is very low if precautions are taken, such as having the appropriate vaccinations (NICE 2018). Routine vaccinations need to be up to date for the specific areas of travel. The GPN will therefore need to advise that the risk of contracting an infectious disease abroad depends on:

- The region visited – the risk may vary from country to country and even areas within countries
- The length of stay – the longer the visit, the greater the risk of exposure
- The time of stay and season of year
- The type of holiday as some areas are riskier than others – for instance, rural areas compared with developed areas
- The age and relative health of the traveller.

The consultation is also an opportunity for general health promotion, such as discussing risky behaviour when abroad and the need for contraception.

Travel health advice and immunisation for travel are not provided in all GP practices. All vaccines for travel can be given in primary care but yellow fever can only be administered at a registered centre. However, it is important for the GPN to understand what these services are, and how they can be accessed. Some vaccines may be provided on the NHS free of charge to patients who require them under some circumstances. These are tetanus, polio, hepatitis A and typhoid. In the case of the hepatitis A and B combination vaccine, NHS patients cannot be charged for hepatitis A where it is required for travel. Patients are therefore not charged for combination hepatitis A and B where indicated for travel. The centrally supplied vaccines for child immunisation should not be used for the supply of travel vaccines. The following vaccines are not available on the NHS: meningitis, tick-borne encephalitis, hepatitis B, Japanese encephalitis, rabies, yellow fever vaccine.

These vaccinations can be obtained in one of two ways:
- By being purchased by the practice and personally administered
- By the practice issuing an FP10 (prescription) and claiming via the prescription pricing division (PPD).

When the patient obtains the vaccination on FP10 prescription, a prescription charge is payable to the pharmacy dispensing the vaccines unless the patient is exempt from medication charges. In this situation no claim for a personal administration fee should be made.

Travel vaccines that are not available on the NHS can be offered to patients as a separate private service. A private prescription can therefore be issued for the patient to take to a pharmacy and practices may charge for this service at their discretion. Alternatively, many practices keep a stock of travel vaccines and may invoice the patient. Not all GP surgeries provide this service. See NICE (2018) for specific information about the different vaccines.

Risk assessment for travel

International travel can pose various risks to health, depending on the health of the traveller and the mode of travel. Any travel health consultation should therefore be treated as an opportunity for health promotion activity. It is not simply a matter of considering the travel destination but, rather, looking at a destination to determine risk. Travellers may be exposed to a variety of risk factors in air travel alone, such as sudden and significant changes in altitude, humidity, microbes or air quality (WHO 2018a). There may also be serious health risks regarding their accommodation, such as poor hygiene and sanitation. It is therefore important to undertake a detailed risk assessment to determine the most significant risks to the individual's health on their overseas trip and this is often part of the GPN's role (Leggat 2006, Zuckerman 2002).

Risk assessment is an integral part of pre-travel and post-travel assessment and determines what health and safety advice and interventions are given to the patient (Leggat 2006). This is because cardiovascular disease and trauma are the most significant causes of death in travellers (Leggat & Fischerb 2006, Steffen *et al.* 2003). Road traffic accidents are a major cause of morbidity and mortality of travellers worldwide (Leggat & Fischerb 2006). We may also have to assess those international travellers with immunocompromising conditions such as human immunodeficiency virus (HIV) infection or solid organ transplantation, as they are at significant risk of communicable and non-communicable diseases which are travel-related, (Aung *et al.* 2015).

International travellers who travel with the specific intention of visiting friends or relatives (Behrens *et al.* 2010) are also at risk of travel-related morbidity or mortality. They often return to see family or friends without considering travel health or vaccinations. This is certainly an increasing risk with the increase in worldwide migration (Zuckerman 2002, WHO 2018b).

It may be worth mentioning here that refugees or migrants are not significantly more vulnerable to mental and physical illness, but they can be exposed to various stress factors (WHO 2018c). They are a vulnerable group who need to be offered appropriate care.

Guidance for prescribers on risk assessment for travellers can be accessed at the National Travel Health Network and Centre website (NaTHNaC).

General travel health

There are a range of resources that we can pass onto our patients, including:

- Guidance on safe food for travellers (WHO 2007)
- The Foreign Office guide to travel to specific countries including information on local laws, travel, terrorism etc. (GOV.UK 2019)
- Fit for Travel provides link to specific organisations about different medical conditions (Health Protection Scotland 2019).

Avoiding mosquito bites

Mosquitoes not only pass on malaria but are also responsible for spreading dengue fever, chikungunya, zika virus and yellow fever.

The type of mosquito that passes on malaria typically bites after sunset. Mosquitoes that bite during the day can transmit other diseases, so it is important to reduce exposure to bites. The following advice about reducing exposure to mosquito bites has been adapted from Fit for Travel (Health Protection Scotland 2019):

- Wear long-sleeved clothing and long trousers to cover the skin
- Spray an insecticide or repellent on clothes as mosquitoes can penetrate thin clothing
- Spray insecticide in the room and use pyrethroid coils or insecticide-impregnated tablets
- Use an impregnated mosquito net
- Use insect repellent on exposed skin such as N,N-Diethyl-m-tolumide (DEET), which is an effective mosquito repellent
- Bear in mind that the duration of protection depends on the concentration:

    20 per cent DEET lasts between 1 and 3 hours

    30 per cent DEET lasts up to 6 hours.

    50 per cent DEET lasts up to 12 hours

    Duration of protection does not increase with concentrations above 50 per cent.

Icaridin (KBR 3023) (1piperidinecarboxylic acid, 2-(2 hydroxyethyl)-,1-methyl-propylester) is also used for mosquito avoidance and is also available in various concentrations. The efficacy of 20 per cent Icaridin is very similar to that of 20 per cent DEET (Frances *et al.* 2004). In fact DEET and Icaridin and ethyl butylacetylaminopropionate (IR3535) have been found to provide protection against mosquitoes but volatile oils and other natural products are less reliable (Goodyer *et al.* 2010).

Please note: Garlic, vitamin B and ultrasound devices do not prevent bites.

Anti-malarial medication

The recommendations on prophylaxis are based on guidelines agreed by UK malaria specialists (PHE 2014). These are specific to the area the patient is travelling to. The GPN has many resources to help patients make an informed decision about anti-malarials, including Fit for Travel (Health Protection Scotland 2019) and BNF (2018) and NICE (2018). Patients should be advised to purchase enough prophylactic medicines to cover the entire period of their travel, including the period prior to travel, while they are abroad and a specified time after their return.

The amount needed depends on the specific medication being used. Most anti-malarials are commenced one week prior to travel, except for mefloquine which should be started two and a half weeks before departure. Patients are advised to take mefloquine for this period in case there are any adverse events that occur prior to travel – to allow time to switch to an alternative medication if necessary before leaving. Most medication needs to be taken for at least four weeks after return.

Malarone is an exception, being started 1–2 days before travel and stopped one week after leaving (BNF 2018). It is also advisable to take anti-malarials at the same time each day (BNF 2018).

Anti-malarials

Atovaquone/Proguanil

Adult dose is one tablet daily – each tablet contains 250mg atovaquone plus 100mg proguanil.

Should be taken to 1 or 2 days before entering the malarious area, throughout exposure, and continued for 7 days after leaving the infected area. It is licensed for periods of up to 28 days. It is also licensed for children over 11kg in weight at a lower dosage and there is a children's tablet available.

Possible side effects: Rashes, abdominal pain, headache, anorexia, nausea, diarrhoea, dizziness, changes in sleep patterns, coughing and mouth ulcers.

Atovaquone/proguanil may interact with other medicines such as tetracyclines and metoclopramide. Proguanil may also interact with warfarin.

Cautions: Patients with kidney disease. This medication should be avoided in pregnancy and breastfeeding unless there is no suitable alternative.

Choloroquine

Adult dose is 2 tablets taken once a week – commonly used brand is Avloclor® (Zeneca). It should be started 1 week before exposure, throughout exposure and for 4 weeks afterwards.

Possible side effects: Nausea, diarrhoea, headache, rashes, skin itch, blurred vision, hair loss, dizziness, mood changes, sun sensitivity or seizures.

Cautions: Antacids should be taken at least 2 hours before or after taking chloroquine. Long- term use of chloroquine can affect the eyes. You need to carefully consider each case if the patient has kidney or liver disease. It can also exacerbate psoriasis and/or those with a history of idiopathic epilepsy should be monitored. Chloroquine is considered to be safe in pregnancy.

Proguanil

The commonest brand is Paludrine® (Zeneca).

Adult dose is 200mg daily which can be used continuously for a maximum of 5 years.
Possible side effects: Anorexia, nausea, diarrhoea, constipation, skin itch and mouth ulcers. It can also alter the metabolism of warfarin.

Caution: Patients with kidney disease. It is, however, safe in pregnancy, but pregnant women should take a folate supplement.

Mefloquine

Adult dose is 250mg week and the brand is known as Lariam®.

One dose should be taken a week before travel, continued throughout exposure and for 4 weeks afterwards. It is, however, advisable to take three doses at weekly intervals prior to departure. This is to ensure that there are no side effects.

Possible side effects: Nausea, diarrhoea, dizziness, abdominal pain, rashes, itch, headache, dizziness, convulsions, sleep disturbances (insomnia, vivid dreams) and psychotic reactions such as depression.

Cautions: Not to be prescribed for patients with a history of severe liver disease, depression, generalised anxiety disorder, psychosis, schizophrenia, suicide attempts, suicidal thoughts, self-endangering behaviour or any other psychiatric disorder, epilepsy or convulsions, or for those with kidney disease or CHD. It should also be avoided during the first trimester of pregnancy.

Doxycycline

Adult dose is 100mg daily. One or two doses should be taken before travel, while abroad and for 4 weeks afterwards.

It should be taken at the same time of day with food.

Possible side effects: Anorexia, nausea, diarrhoea, thrush, sore tongue (glossitis), headaches, blurred vision or tinnitus. Erythema (sunburn) due to sunlight photosensitivity; sunscreens are important and, if severe, alternative anti-malarials should be used.

Cautions: There is the potential for drug interactions with iron or zinc tablets, retinoids or cyclosporine. Phenytoin, barbiturates and carbamazapine may reduce the efficacy of the doxycycline. It is also contraindicated in pregnancy.

Adapted from Fit for Travel (Health Protection Scotland 2019)

Box 8.1: Anti-malarials

Other medication

Patients can take out medications which are prescribed in anticipation of illness whilst abroad. An example of this is ciprofloxacin, which is used for traveller's diarrhoea. Patients leaving the UK for more than three months should be advised to register with a local doctor for their continuing medical needs. Patients can request a three-month supply of their medication from their GP. It is advisable that patients travelling with medication in their hand luggage should have a covering letter from their GP.

Please note: Some countries have their own import regulations. It is therefore advisable for travellers to contact the country's embassy to check prior to travel.

Summary

We have discussed the fact that travel advice, risk assessment and travel vaccinations can be complicated and the GPN who is involved in this aspect of care needs to have extensive training and keep up to date (Zuckerman 2002). A range of resources are listed in this chapter to help and support the GPN in this role. There is both general advice and health promotion but also advice that is specific to an area, country or if the patient has specific conditions. Recommendations on general travel advice can be accessed in the Green Book (PHE 2014) and from the National Travel Health Network and Centre (NaTHNaC) and the Travel HealthPro website (NaTHNaC).

Resources

BNF/NICE malarial prophylaxis: https://bnf.nice.org.uk/treatment-summary/malaria-prophylaxis.html

National Travel Health Network and Centre website (NaTHNaC): https://nathnac.net/

PHE (2014). The Green Book: https://www.gov.uk/government/collections/immunisation-against-infectious-disease-the-green-book

WHO international travel health updates: http://www.who.int/ith/en/

Box 8.2: Resources

References

Aung, A.K., Trubiano, J.A. & Spelman, D.W. (2015). Travel risk assessment, advice and vaccinations in immunocompromised travellers (HIV, solid organ transplant and haematopoietic stem cell transplant recipients): a review. *Travel Medicine and Infectious Disease.* **13**(1), 31–47.

Behrens, R.H., Stauffer, W.M., Barnett, E.D., Loutan, L., Hatz, C.F., Matteelli, A. & MacPherson, D.W. (2010). Travel case scenarios as a demonstration of risk assessment of VFR travelers: introduction to criteria and evidence-based definition and framework. *Journal of Travel Medicine.* **17**(3), 153–62.

British National Formulary (BNF) (2018). *Treatment summary for antimalarials.* https://bnf.nice.org.uk/treatment-summary/antimalarials.html (last accessed 17.1.2019).

Frances, S.P., Waterson, D.G.E., Beebe, N.W. & Cooper, R. D. (2004). Field evaluation of repellent formulations containing DEET and picaridin against mosquitoes in Northern Territory, Australia. *Journal of Medical Entomology.* **41**(3), 414–17.

Goodyer, L.I., Croft, A.M., Frances, S.P., Hill, N., Moore, S.J., Onyango, S. P. & Debboun, M. (2010). Expert review of the evidence base for arthropod bite avoidance. *Journal of Travel Medicine.* **17**(3), 182–92.

GOV.UK (2019). https://www.gov.uk/foreign-travel-advice (last accessed 17.1.2019).

Health Protection Scotland (2019). https://www.fitfortravel.nhs.uk/resources/specialist-associations (last accessed 16.1.2019).

Leggat, P.A. (2006). Risk assessment in travel medicine. *Travel Medicine and Infectious Disease.* **4**(3–4), 127–34.

Leggat, P.A. & Fischerb, P. (2006). Accidents and repatriation. *Travel Medicine and Infectious Disease.* **4** (3–4), 135–46.

National Travel Health Network and Centre website (NaTHNaC) https://nathnac.net/ (last accessed 16.1.2019).

National Travel Health Network and Centre website (NaTHNaC) https://travelhealthpro.org.uk/ (last accessed 17.1.2019).

NICE (2018). *Immunizations.* https://cks.nice.org.uk/immunizations-travel (last accessed 17.1.2019).

Public Health England (PHE) (2014). *Immunisation against infectious disease – the Green Book.* https://www.gov.uk/government/collections/immunisation-against-infectious-disease-the-green-book (last accessed 17.1.2019).

Steffen, R., deBernardis, C. & Banos, A. (2003). Travel epidemiology – a global perspective. *International Journal of Antimicrobial Agents.* **21**, 89–95.

World Health Organization (WHO) (2017). http://www.who.int/foodsafety/publications/consumer/en/travellers_en.pdf?ua=1 (last accessed 17.1.2019).

World Health Organization (WHO) (2018a). *Travel health.* http://www.who.int/topics/travel/en/ (last accessed 17.1.2019).

World Health Organization (WHO) (2018b). *Migration.* http://www.who.int/hrh/migration/en/ (last accessed 17.1.2019).

World Health Organization (WHO) (2018c). *Refugee and migrant health.* http://www.who.int/migrants/about/areas-of-work/en/index5.html (last accessed 17.1.2019).

Zuckerman, J.N. (2002). Recent developments: travel medicine. *British Medical Journal.* **325**(7358), 260.

Chapter 9

Ear care

Sian Hayes and Deborah Duncan

Introduction

There are different views on how and when ear irrigation should be performed. For most people, ear wax is a healthy positive thing. We would suggest that nurses undertaking ear syringing first undergo appropriate training, or they should refer patients to an ENT clinic to have the procedure carried out (Rotherham Primary Ear Care Centre and Audiology Services 2016).

The pros and cons of ear wax removal

The consensus of opinion is that we currently syringe too much (Rotherham Primary Ear Care Centre and Audiology Services 2016). In one study about 44,000 ears were syringed by 312 general practitioners serving a population of about 650,000 (Sharpe *et al.* 1990). This research showed that the incidence of complications could be reduced by a greater awareness of the potential hazards, increased patient education and appropriate clients (ibid.). We know that alleged iatrogenic injuries following ear syringing can account for about 25 per cent of medical negligence claims (Blake *et al.* 1998).

Ear wax should therefore only be removed if:

- It is affecting hearing (think impacted wax and features of conductive hearing loss)
- It is preventing visualisation of the ear drum which is necessary for diagnosis
- Removal is necessary in order to make moulds for hearing aids.

In fact, Rotherham Primary Ear Care Centre and Audiology Services (2016) suggest that ear removal should only be considered:
- For removal of debris following otitis media/otitis externa
- To improve the conduction of sound to the tympanic membrane (TM) when it is obscured by wax
- To remove discharge, keratin or debris to allow examination of the external auditory meatus
- To remove wax prior to hearing aid mould impressions being taken
- To facilitate the removal of wax and foreign bodies, which are not hygroscopic, from the external auditory meatus
- For removal of hygroscopic matter (such as lentils and cotton wool) that will absorb the water and expand, making them more difficult to remove.

NICE (2016) suggest that we should remove ear wax if it is blocking the ear canal and/or any of the following conditions are present:
- Hearing loss
- Earache
- Tinnitus
- Vertigo
- Cough suspected to be due to ear wax
- If the tympanic membrane is obscured by wax but needs to be viewed to establish a diagnosis
- If the person wears a hearing aid, wax is present and an impression needs to be taken of the ear canal for a mould, or if wax is causing the hearing aid to whistle.

Self-care by patients

What is recommended is to encourage self-care by patients (NICE 2016, Schwartz *et al.* 2017). There is evidence that oiling and self-irrigation can work well for a significant number of patients (NICE 2016). One suggestion is that each practice should produce a leaflet encouraging patients to use self-care, before accessing ear irrigation with the nurse. Patients should be encouraged to oil their ears, using a softening agent (such as olive oil), and then book an appointment for irrigation of their ear(s) if it is still required (Clegg *et al.* 2010). You also need to ensure there are no contraindications prior to undertaking the procedure. Furthermore, it is recommended not to use cotton buds as patients can end up pushing the wax further into the canal, causing it to become compacted (Adegbiji *et al.* 2014).

Self-management

NICE provides the following advice on self-management:

- Prescribe ear drops for 3–5 days initially, to soften wax and aid removal
- Olive oil or almond oil drops can be used 3–4 times daily for 3–5 days (do not prescribe almond oil ear drops to anyone who is allergic to almonds)
- Sodium bicarbonate 5 per cent, sodium chloride 0.9 per cent (sodium chloride 0.9 per cent is not available as a proprietary ear drop product but sodium chloride 0.9 per cent nasal drops can be prescribed for off-label use in the ear)
- Do not prescribe drops if you suspect the person has a perforated tympanic membrane
- Warn the person that instilling ear drops may cause transient hearing loss, discomfort, dizziness and irritation of the skin.

Box 9.1: Self-management ear care advice (NICE 2016)

If the problem has not been resolved using these measures, the patient can attend their GP practice to have their ear syringed or be referred to a local ENT clinic. If ear irrigation is unsuccessful, there are three options:

- Advise the person to use ear drops for a further 3–5 days and then return for further irrigation
- Instil warm water into the ear; after 15 minutes irrigate the ear again
- Refer to an ENT specialist for removal of wax.

Main methods of wax removal

There are three strategies for removal, none of which are supported by a strong evidence base (NICE, 2016). If using an ear syringe for irrigation, the equipment of choice is the Propulse II, III, NG, or G5 irrigators (NICE 2016, Rotherham Primary Ear Care Centre and Audiology Services 2016). This is because they have a pressure-variable control so the flow of water can easily be controlled and irrigation can be started on the minimum setting (Rotherham Primary Ear Care Centre and Audiology Services 2016). Find out what equipment you have in your own practice and read the instructions carefully.

If your patient does not respond to the combination of ear drops and irrigation, or if these are contraindicated, they may need to have the following procedures done

at a specialist centre or by a GP with a special interest in ENT:
- Microsuction – a gentle level of suction is used to remove the wax from the ear
- Aural toilet: a Jobson–Horne probe is used to remove the wax.

(Adapted from NICE 2016)

Table 9.1: Methods of ear wax removal

Method	Any wax softener has been shown to be better than no treatment None is superior	Irrigation with motorised pump Only weak evidence that using wax softeners beforehand improves outcomes	Binocular microscopes with an otoendoscope are safest but expensive training for their use is required
When to use	First line in primary care where no contraindications	Second line in primary care where no contraindications	Chronic perforation Previous ear surgery Persistent otitis externa People with pre-existing hearing loss in one ear
Harms	Failure of treatment Otitis externa	Risk of perforation, vertigo and tinnitus Otitis externa Rarely deafness	Damage to ear canal

(Adapted from Rotherham Primary Ear Care Centre and Audiology Services 2016)

In most cases, the wax usually falls out on its own but, if it doesn't, softening the wax twice a day, for at least five days, may speed up the process. Patients may find some of the wax falls out, especially at night when they are lying down.

Ear candles

One popular procedure is ear candling even though there is absolutely no evidence that it is effective. Ear candles are hollow tubes that are coated in wax. They are inserted into patients' ears and then lit at the far end. A critical assessment of the evidence shows no data to suggest that this method is effective for removing any compacted ear wax (Ernst 2004). Certainly, the mechanism of the action has not been verified and it appears to have no positive clinical effect at all (Rafferty 2006).

> *Reader activity*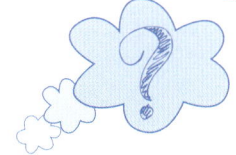
>
> List the main reasons for ear syringing, according to NICE (2016).

Box 9.3: Reader activity – ear syringing (answers on p. 82)

The potential complications of ear syringing

The following complications have been reported following ear syringing:

- Failure to remove ear wax
- Otitis externa
- Perforation of the tympanic membrane
- Damage to the external auditory meatus
- Pain
- Vertigo
- Otitis media due to water entering the middle ear when there is a pre-existing perforation
- Exacerbation of pre-existing tinnitus
- Bleeding may also occur but is usually self-limiting
- Nausea, vomiting and vertigo may result from the temperature variations of the irrigating fluid.

Legal implications

As GPNs, we have a legal duty of care to our patients, but we also follow the common law of negligence and the civil law. Patients may therefore claim compensation if there is a complication during the procedure. If the nurse is guilty of professional misconduct, whether or not the patient has suffered harm, the nurse may also face misconduct proceedings before the NMC's professional conduct committee.

Reader activity

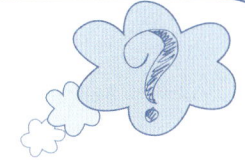

List the main reasons for ear syringing.
- Hearing loss
- Earache
- Tinnitus
- Vertigo
- Cough suspected to be due to ear wax
- If the tympanic membrane is obscured by wax but needs to be viewed to establish a diagnosis
- If the person wears a hearing aid, wax is present and an impression needs to be taken of the ear canal for a mould, or if wax is causing the hearing aid to whistle.

Box 9.4: Answers to reader activity – ear syringing

Resources

NICE provides the following advice on self-management:
NHS: https://www.nhs.uk/conditions/earwax-build-up/
NICE (2016): https://cks.nice.org.uk/earwax
RCN competencies – An education and training framework for aural care nursing and treatment provision: https://www.rcn.org.uk/professional-development/publications/pdf-006855
Rotherham Primary Ear Care Centre and Audiology Services 2016: https://www.guidelinesfornurses.co.uk/RotherhamNHSFT/Ear-irrigation/452732.article

Box 9.5: Resources

References

Adegbiji, W., Alabi, B., Olajuyin, O. & Nwawolo, C. (2014). Earwax impaction: Symptoms, predisposing factors and perception among Nigerians. *Journal of Family Medicine and Primary Care.* (4), 379–82. doi: 10.4103/2249-4863.148116.

Blake, P., Matthews, R. & Hornibrook, J. (1998). When not to syringe an ear. *The New Zealand Medical Journal.* **111**(1077), 422–24.

Clegg, A.J., Loveman, E., Gospodarevskaya, E., Harris, P., Bird, A., Bryant, J., Scott, D.A., Davidson, P., Little. P. & Coppin, R. (2010). The safety and effectiveness of different methods of earwax removal: a systematic review and economic evaluation. *Health Technology Assessment.* **14**(28), 1–192. doi: 10.3310/hta14280.

Ernst, E. (2004). Ear candles: a triumph of ignorance over science. *The Journal of Laryngology & Otology.* **118**(1), 1–2.

NICE (2016). *Ear wax.* https://cks.nice.org.uk/earwax#!scenario (last accessed 19.1.2019).

Rafferty, J., Tsikoudas, A. & Davis, B. C. (2007). Ear candling: should general practitioners recommend it? *Canadian Family Physician.* **53**(12), 2121–22.

Rotherham Primary Ear Care Centre and Audiology Services (2016). *Ear irrigation guideline. Rotherham NHS Foundation Trust.* https://www.guidelinesfornurses.co.uk/RotherhamNHSFT/Ear-irrigation/452732.article (last accessed 19.1.2019).

Schwartz, S., Magit, A.E., Rosenfeld, R., Ballachanda, B., Hackell, J., Krouse, H., Lawlor, C., Lin, K., Parham, K., Stutz, D., Walsh, S., Woodson, E., Yanagisawa, K. & Cunningham, E. (2017). Clinical Practice Guideline (Update): Earwax (Cerumen Impaction). *Otolaryngology–Head and Neck Surgery.* **156**(1), S1–S29. doi: 10.1177/0194599816671491.

Sharp, J.F., Wilson, J.A., Ross, L. & Barr-Hamilton, R.M. (1990). Ear wax removal: a survey of current practice. *British Medical Journal.* **301**(6763), 1251–53.

Chapter 10
Wound care

Nuala McCarron

Introduction

General Practice Nurses will encounter a wide variety of wounds in their everyday practice. This can be both complex and challenging. Our ever-growing elderly population, living with multiple comorbidities, are at increasing risk of developing a wound. They also tend to develop many complex wounds as a result of multiple comorbidities (NHS England 2014). The cost of chronic wounds is set to increase exponentially with a growing elderly population (NICE 2016). The findings of Guest *et al.* (2015) highlighted the need for change and this was actioned by the inclusion of wound assessment as a key indicator in the Commissioning for Quality and Innovation Framework (CQUIN) for 2017–19 (NHS England 2019).

The function of the skin

The skin is the largest organ of the body and makes up 16 per cent of body weight. Its main functions include: playing a role in the immune system, temperature regulation, sensation and vitamin production. The skin is also a dynamic organ, in a constant state of change, as the outer layers are continuously shed and replaced by inner cells which migrate to the surface. The main layers are: the epidermis, the dermis and the hypodermis.

The epidermis is the outer layer of the skin and is composed of epithelial cells which are avascular cells, 0.04mm thick and are regenerated every 2–4 weeks. They are fed by nutrients from the dermis layer below.

The dermis is the middle layer of the skin and is 1.5 to 4 mm thick, depending on which bony structure it is covering. It is a vascular layer and contains nerves, connective tissue, collagen, elastin and specialised cells such as fibroblasts and mast cells. It is mainly responsible for inflammatory reactions and also contains receptors for sensations such as heat, cold, pain, pressure, itch and tickle.

The hypodermis is the innermost layer of the skin and supports the dermis and epidermis. This layer varies in thickness and depth and is composed of adipose tissue, connective tissue and blood vessels. Its main functions are: to store lipids, protect the underlying organs and provide insulation and regulate the body's temperature.

Defining types of wounds

Wounds generally occur when there is trauma, infection or when the skin is cut or broken. Acute wounds may include post-surgical, skin tears, lacerations, bites or burns. They will usually heal fast, varying from 5 to 15 days, depending on their location and depth (Chester & Brown 2017).

Chronic wounds, such as diabetic foot ulcers, pressure ulcers and leg ulcers, have generally been present for 4 to 6 or more weeks and 'normal' wound healing has been disrupted. If it is a recurring wound or has an underlying comorbidity, it can be considered chronic from as early as 2 weeks (NICE 2016).

Holistic assessment of wounds is therefore essential, coupled with a sound understanding of the principles of wound healing and a knowledge of the intervention/dressing required. In order to provide high-quality wound care, it is essential for health professionals to be equipped with the knowledge and skills that will help them undertake this challenging role (Newton 2017).

Wound healing

Wounds heal in two main ways, known as primary and secondary intention.

Primary intention involves the edges of the wound being brought together, using sutures, staples or clips.

Secondary intention occurs when there is a large amount of tissue loss. The wound heals by the formation of granulation tissue and epithelisation.

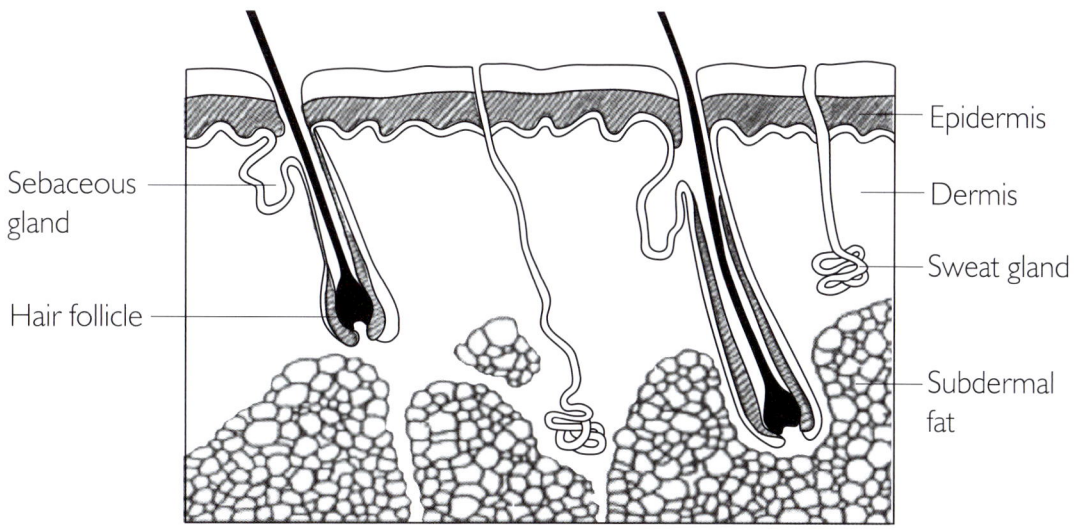

Figure 10.1: Layers of the skin

There are many models of wound healing, but we are going to focus on the four stages approach, which includes inflammation, destruction, proliferation and maturation (Chester & Brown 2017). These are outlined below.

Phase 1: Inflammation – the fire fighters

This phase starts immediately after the injury is caused and lasts 0–3 days (Nguyen *et al.* 2009). It is the body's emergency response to the injury. Once bleeding has stopped, the blood vessels dilate, and redness, heat, swelling and pain are present. This is caused by the action of histamine and prostaglandins at the wound site.

Phase 2: Destruction – the refuse collectors

The destructive phase lasts 1–6 days. Once a house fire has been extinguished, the refuse collectors come in to clean up the debris. Similarly, within a wound, the destructive phase prevents infection, cleans the wound and provides the best conditions for healing to occur (Li *et al.* 2007). White blood cells enter the wound and digest bacteria. When the bacteria and the white cells die off, they can be seen as moist sticky tissue, known as slough (Wolcott *et al.* 2008).

Phase 3: Proliferation – the builders

After the debris from a house fire has been cleared, builders are called in to restore the house. In wound healing this is the proliferation phase, which usually lasts 3–24 days. Tiny new capillaries join to form a scaffold within the wound. This develops into granulation tissue which fills the wound cavity (Martin 2013).

Phase 4: Maturation – the decorators

The maturation phase can be likened to redecorating the house after a fire. It lasts between 21 days and 2 years. Epithelial cells, located in intact hair follicles, sweat glands and around the edges of the wound, move over the newly formed granulation tissues and reduce the size of the wound.

Wound assessment

Improving the assessment of wounds is the tenth of 13 national indicators. The aim is to reduce the number of wounds which have failed to heal after 4 weeks of treatment by focusing on wound assessment (Wounds UK 2008). A holistic patient assessment is essential in order to identify the causative or contributing factors that could potentially delay or prevent wound healing (Wounds UK 2008). Both intrinsic and extrinsic factors affect wound healing and it is vital that all these factors are considered as part of the holistic assessment. Any risk factors that could result in delayed healing (whether intrinsic or extrinsic) should be considered, identified and eliminated or optimally managed where possible (Chamanga 2016). See the summary in Table 10.1 below.

Table 10.1: Factors that affect wound healing *(Adapted from Chester & Brown 2017).*

INTRINSIC	EXTRINSIC
Health status: Good blood supply or oxygenation	Physical damage: • Pressure • Friction • Shearing forces
Immune function: • Helps the wound healing process • Reduces the risk of wound infection	Debris: • Slough • Necrotic tissue • Eschar • Scab
Comorbidities: • Diabetes • Autoimmune disease • Pain (increases the production of cortisol)	Desiccation: • Drying of wound surface resulting in death of surface cells
Age-related skin changes: • Loss of hair follicles, receptors, sweat glands • Reduced blood supply • Increased fragility • Dryness/thinning	Maceration: • Excess exudate • Temperature

Nutrition:	Infection:
• A balanced diet including proteins for the amino acid arginine, carbohydrates, fats and fluids promote healing	• Chemical stresses may have an adverse effect • Topical agents such as antiseptics • Smoking • Steroids and non-steroidal anti-inflammatory drugs

The GPN also needs to undertake a full assessment of the wound. All patients presenting with either new or recurrent leg ulceration should have a complete clinical history and physical examination, which should include screening for evidence of arterial disease by measurement of Ankle Bracial Pressure Index (ABPI) using a Doppler (NICE 2018).

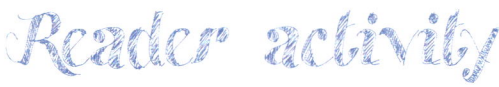 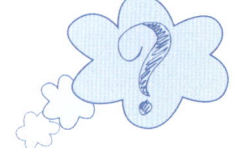

Arterial and venous ulcers
Review your local policy on the care of arterial and venous leg ulcers in your area of practice. Discuss this with your mentor.

Box 10.1: Reader activity – ulcers

A helpful acronym for wound assessment is **BESSSOP** (Health & Social Care 2011):

Bed – one of the most effective ways of describing the tissue type is by its colour:

- Black – necrotic/eschar
- Yellow – sloughy
- Red – granulating
- Pink – epithelialising.

Exudate – knowing the level and type of wound exudate is extremely important as this will influence dressing choice.
The level of exudate may be described as:

- Dry – no exudate
- Low – the wound bed is moist
- Moderate – the surrounding skin is wet
- High – the surrounding skin is macerated and the wound is bathed in fluid.

The type may be described as:
- Serous – clear fluid
- Sanguinous – bloody
- Serosanguinous – blood mixed with clear fluid
- Purulent – pus-like, cloudy yellow.

Site is important to describe, as it:
- Differentiates between wounds
- Position of wound may indicate aetiology.

Size – accurate size is vital for assessing the progress of healing. For all wounds, you should carry out a two-dimensional assessment of the wound opening and a three-dimensional assessment of any cavity or tracking (Carville *et al.* 2007).

A two-dimensional measure can be taken using a paper tape to measure the length and width of the wound. The circumference of the wound can be traced if the wound edges are not even. A three-dimensional measure should be performed to assess the wound depth, using a dampened cotton tip applicator.

Methods therefore include:
- Ruler-based transparency
- Transparency
- Photography with written informed consent
- Cotton tip applicator.

The surrounding skin provides important information about underlying disease and the effectiveness of the treatment regime, e.g. pink/purple tissue on the edges of the wound may indicate epithelialisation, while maceration may indicate an ineffective dressing regime.

Odour may be caused by infection, necrotic tissue or certain dressings. The cause must be identified and (where possible) rectified.

Pain is subjective but its location, frequency and severity can be helpful in determining the presence of underlying disease or infection, the exposure of nerve endings, the efficiency of wound dressing and psychological need. Visual or verbal rating scales may be used.

Table 10.2: Exudate

Type	Colour	Consistency	Significance
Serous	Clear, straw-coloured	Thin and watery	Normal but monitor the amount, as it may indicate infection if it increases
Haemoserous	Clear, pink	Thin and watery	Normal
Sanguinous	Bright red	Thin and watery	There is trauma to blood vessels
Purulent	Yellow, grey, green	Thick	Infection, as there are pyogenic organisms and other inflammatory cells

Selecting a dressing

The GPN needs to understand the principles of wound healing prior to selecting a dressing. Evidence shows us that a moist wound environment is essential for wound healing (NICE 2016). Certainly, the dressings should provide the optimal environment for wound healing but choosing the correct dressing may be difficult and confusing, as there are so many different dressings available (NICE 2016). The final choice of dressing will depend on:

- The stage of wound healing
- The amount of exudate
- If there is evidence of infection
- The odour
- The adhesiveness of a dressing for ease of removal
- If there is any irritation caused by the adhesive
- How absorbent the dressing is
- The frequency of dressing changes required
- The ease of use of the dressing
- The amount of pain at dressing changes
- How much of the surrounding skin needs to be protected
- Patient preference.

Working in a wound dressing formulary is a way of directing wound care interventions and the effective prescription of wound dressings (Cryer 2015). Table 10.3 details some of the dressing types that are currently available.

Table 10.3: Dressing selection *(Adapted from Baranoski & Ayello, 2008)*

Dressing type	Description	Indications
Transparent film	Polyurethane or co-polymer with porous adhesive layer that varies in thickness and allows oxygen to pass through the membrane and moisture vapour to escape	• Donor sites • Primary and secondary dressings • Partial thickness wounds • Pressure ulcers, grade 1 and 2 • Superficial burns • Abrasions
Hydrocolloid	Hydrophilic colloid particles bound in polyurethane foam	• Pressure ulcers grade 1–4 • Partial and full thickness wounds • Under compression • Necrotic wounds
Hydrogel	Water- or glycerine-based, non-adhesive, cross-linked polymer	• Pressure ulcers grade 2–4 • Partial and full thickness wounds • Painful wounds • Radiation tissue damage • Minor burns • Donor sites • Necrotic wounds
Hydrofibre	Made from sodium carboxymethyl-cellulose that interacts with wound exudate to form a gel	• Partial and full thickness wounds • Moderate to heavy exuding wounds • Pressure ulcers grade 3 and 4 • Surgical wounds • Donor sites • Sinus tracts, tunnels, cavities
Calcium alginate	Non-woven composite of fibres from calcium sodium alginate, highly absorptive dressing manufactured from brown seaweed	• Partial and full thickness wounds with moderate to heavy exudate • Pressure ulcers grade 3 and 4 • Surgical wounds • Donor sites • Sinus tracts, tunnels, cavities • Infected wounds
Foam	Hydrophilic polyurethane or gel film-coated foam, non-occulusive, non-adherent layer absorptive dressing	• Partial and full thickness wounds with minimal to heavy exudate • Pressure ulcers grade 2–4 • Surgical wounds • Under compression
Composites	Combination of two or more physically distinct products manufactured as a single dressing that provides multiple functions	• Primary and secondary dressings for partial and full thickness wounds • Pressure ulcers grade 1–4 • Minimal to heavily exuding wounds

Wound care

Antimicrobial	Non-adherent that protects against bacteria and/or decreases bacterial load	• Infected wounds • Partial and full thickness wounds • Colonised non-healing wounds
Silver	Immediate and sustained release of ionic silver, effective barrier to bacterial penetration	• Infected wounds • Highly colonised wounds, except grade 1 pressure ulcers, third degree burns and non-exuding wounds under pressure

Infection

All open wounds are colonised but bacteriological culture is indicated only if clinical signs of infection are present or if infection control issues, such as methicillin-resistant staphylococcus aureus (MRSA), need to be considered. Most community wound care involves managing chronic wounds where identifying the wound infection can be challenging for a clinician. The classic signs of infection are heat, redness, swelling and pain. Additional signs of wound infection include increased exudate, delayed healing, contact bleeding, odour and abnormal granulation tissue. Treatment with antimicrobials should be guided by microbiological results and local resistance patterns (Grey *et al.* 2006). To provide effective, evidence-based and cost-efficient care, the GPN needs an understanding of the more commonly used antimicrobial treatments in the local area and when to initiate treatment supports (Rutter 2018).

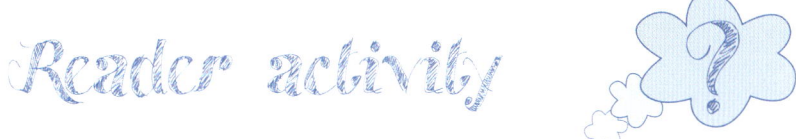

Wound infection
List the main signs and symptoms of a wound infection.

Box 10.2: Reader activity – wound infection (answers on p. 93)

Summary

Nurses in general practice will encounter many different types of wounds. Whatever type of wound management is required, it is crucial to provide patient-centred care. Holistic assessment is essential prior to an evidence-based intervention. The GPN also needs to be able to evaluate care and decide whether to refer the patient to specialist services such as Tissue Viability, Podiatry or the vascular team. These are all fundamental skills for effective wound management.

> **Resources**
> **Advanced wound dressings BNF:** https://bnf.nice.org.uk/wound-management/advanced-wound-dressings.html
> **Wound Care Alliance UK:** https://www.wcauk.org/
> Always review your local guidelines.

Box 10.3: Resources

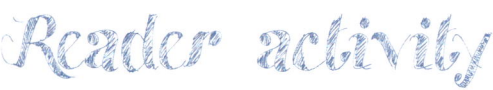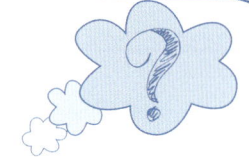

Wound infection
The main signs and symptoms of a wound infection are:
- Redness (erythema or cellulitis) around the wound
- Increased amounts of exudate
- Change in the colour of the exudate
- Malodour/Smell
- Localised pain
- Localised heat
- Delayed or abnormal healing
- Wound breakdown.

Box 10.4: Answers to reader activity – wound infection

References

Baranoski, S. & Ayello, E.A. (2008). *Wound care essentials: Practice principles*. Lippincott Williams & Wilkins.

Carville, K., Lewin, G., Newall, N., Haslehurst, P., Michael, R., Santamaria, N. & Roberts, P. (2007). STAR: a consensus for skin tear classification. *Primary Intention: The Australian Journal of Wound Management*. **15**(1), 18.

Chamanga, E. (2016). Wound assessment and treatment in primary care. *Independent Nurse*. 2016 (5), 18–23.

Chester, D. & Brown, A. C. (2017). The role of biophysical properties of provisional matrix proteins in wound repair. *Matrix Biology*. **60**, 124–40.

Cryer, S. (2015). Improving the selection of wound dressings in general practice. *Nurse Prescribing*. **13**(7), 336–42.

Grey, J.E., Harding, K.G. & Enoch, S. (2006). Venous and arterial leg ulcers. *British Medical Journal*. **332**(7537), 347–50.

Guest, J.F., Ayoub, N., McIlwraith, T., Uchegbu, I., Gerrish, A., Weidlich, D. & Vowden, P. (2015). Health economic burden that wounds impose on the National Health Service in the UK. *British Medical Journal* open. **5**(12), e009283.

Health and Social Care (2011). *Northern Ireland Wound Care Formulary*. 2nd edn. April 2011. http://niformulary.hscni.net/Formulary/Adult/WoundSection/Pages/default.aspx (last accessed 21.1.2019).

Martin, M. (2013). Physiology of wound healing. In Flanagan, M. (ed.) *Wound healing and skin integrity: Principles and practice*. Chichester: Wiley-Blackwell.

Newton, H. (2017). Cost-effective wound management: a survey of 1717 nurses. *British Journal of Nursing*. **26**(12), S44–S49.

Nguyen, D.T., Orgill, D.P. & Murphy, G.T. (2009). '4 The Pathophysiologic Basis for Wound Healing and Cutaneous Regeneration' in D.P. Orgill & C. Blanco (eds) *Biomaterials for Treating Skin Loss*. Elsevier. pp. 25–57.

NHS England (2014) *Five Year Forward View*. [Online] http://www.england.nhs.uk/wp-content/uploads/2014/10/5yfv-web.pdf (last accessed 21.1.2019).

NHS England (2019). https://www.england.nhs.uk/nhs-standard-contract/cquin/cquin-17-19/ (last accessed 5.2.2019).

NICE (2016). *Chronic wounds: advanced wound dressings and antimicrobial dressings. Evidence summary [ESMPB2]*. https://www.nice.org.uk/advice/esmpb2/chapter/Key-points-from-the-evidence (last accessed 21.1.2019).

NICE (2018). *Peripheral arterial disease: diagnosis and management. Clinical guideline [CG147]*. https://www.nice.org.uk/guidance/cg147 (last accessed 21.1.2019).

Rutter, L. (2018). Identifying and managing wound infection in the community. *British Journal of Community Nursing*. **23**(3), S6–S14.

Shaw, T.J. & Martin, P. (2016). Wound repair: a showcase for cell plasticity and migration. *Current Opinion in Cell Biology*. **42**, 29–37.

Wounds UK (2008). *Best practice statement: optimising wound care*. Aberdeen: Wounds UK.

Chapter 11

General principles of long-term conditions

Deborah Duncan

Introduction

Long-term conditions (LTCs), otherwise known as chronic conditions, are conditions for which there is no cure (King's Fund 2018). Although they cannot be cured, they are managed using pharmacological and non-pharmacological methods. Examples of long-term conditions include asthma, diabetes, hypothyroidism and HIV. In the UK there are approximately 15 million people with a long-term condition (DH 2012a). The number is increasing, with some people having two or more conditions (DH 2012a). By 2034, it is predicted that there will be over 3.5 million people aged 85 and over, who will account for 5 per cent of the UK's population (DH 2012a). Many of these elderly people will have at least one LTC and around 15 per cent of young adults have a long-term condition (NHS England 2018).

The main risk factors for developing a long-term condition are lifestyle and ageing. Prevention is therefore very important. The aim is to delay onset and slow down the progression of the disease. These objectives are delivered through public health, personalised patient care planning and supported self-care. People with LTCs continue to be the most intensive users of the most expensive services within the NHS (DH 2012a). The predicted increase in cost to the NHS and social care services, due to increased comorbidities, is likely to be £5 billion in 2018, compared to 2011 (DH 2012).

However, prevention doesn't only matter in terms of cutting costs; it is also important for people's quality of life.

Quality of life

Having an LTC affects all aspects of physical and mental wellbeing. People with LTCs are more likely to experience psychological problems, reduced immunity and the complications of their condition. We know that approximately 30 per cent of all people with an LTC also have a mental health problem such as depression and/or anxiety (Barnett *et al.* 2012). Of those with an LTC, nearly 50 per cent report moderate or extreme pain, rising to 80 per cent of people with three or more conditions (DH 2012a). People living with a long-term condition are also more likely to be disadvantaged in employment, educational opportunities, home ownership and earning power. Certainly, their quality of life is seriously affected and they need a lot of support to help them manage their condition.

Aspects of self-care

The following are the common core self-care tasks in long-term conditions:
- Recognising and responding to symptoms
- Use of medication
- Management of acute episodes/exacerbations
- Managing nutrition, diet and exercise
- Smoking cessation
- Relaxation and stress reduction strategies
- Interacting with healthcare provider
- Use of the community resources
- Managing and adapting to work
- Managing relations with significant others
- Managing emotions.

Box 11.1: Aspects of self-care

Self-care

Dr Michael Dixon, Chair of the NHS Alliance for the DH (2012a) report, said, 'The most crucial issue in the management of long-term conditions is how we better support people to self-care'. He suggested that this would mean empowering patients to manage their own conditions and would also help the NHS control its finances better.

Self-care and better LTC management will also help to narrow the health inequalities gap, which is a key aspect of the Public Health Agenda. In general, people in social class V (the most unskilled working class) have a 60 per cent higher prevalence of long-term conditions and 30 per cent higher severity of conditions than those in the higher socioeconomic classes (DH 2012a). Self-care is about individual behaviour and should consider issues such as health literacy, health-promoting behaviours, self-care, chronic disease self-management, and more social and collective forms of self-care (Cayton 2006). Box 11.1 (above) summarises all aspects of self-care. Primary care is seen as the best context in which to deliver care for people with long-term conditions because it is easily accessible (Kennedy *et al.* 2013).

Self-management

Self-management support is about encouraging patients in their ability to increase their confidence and efficacy in self-management (Kennedy *et al.* 2013). Although the terms 'self-care' and 'self-management' sound interchangeable, they have quite different meanings (Parsons *et al.* 2010).

There are two main forms of self-management. This first is a provider-based model where support is embedded in general nursing care; the second is a patient-based model that enables patients to improve their self-management through individual or group-based education (Kennedy *et al.* 2007). Both approaches have pros and cons. Educational programmes, such as the UK Expert Patients Programme, are utilised, with participants in these programmes being found to be more educated than the general population of patients with LTCs (Lorig *et al.* 2008, Williams *et al.* 2011). Embedding self-management support programmes into everyday practice may work more effectively but can be time-consuming (Ryan *et al.* 2008). Ultimately, supporting self-management is considered as essential as high-quality care for patients with LTCs (Taylor *et al.* 2014).

Any self-management should be tailored to the individual, taking into account their culture and health beliefs. It needs to be underpinned by a collaborative, communicative relationship between the patient and healthcare professionals (Barlow *et al.* 2002, Taylor *et al.* 2014).

Self-management support is a complex intervention and its core components include:
- Specific education about the LTC which considers the patient's knowledge and beliefs about their LTC
- Psychological strategies supporting life and LTC
- Strategies that support concordance to treatments
- Practical support tailored to the specific LTC, such as recognition and treatment of exacerbations
- Social support.

Personalised care planning

Personalised care planning involves patients in the decision-making process about their care. The key message about this is that patient involvement should be the norm (DH 2012b). They are given the information they need to help them make those decisions. This is the key message from the DH (2012b) report, *Liberating the NHS: no decision about me without me.* We should therefore be working within a culture in primary care that supports patient involvement and shared decision-making (King's Fund 2011).

Part of your role as a GPN will be to facilitate the development of personalised care plans for your patients. A care plan records the outcome of discussions between the patient and healthcare professionals and is owned by the individual patient. It contains all the information they need to manage their own care, including their specific concerns, actions, goals, and any particular needs they may have.

Action plans

An action plan, which is specific and focused, is a written set of instructions that is given to the patient (or parent of a child patient). The action plan:
- Is kept by the patient until the next appointment
- Provides instructions for daily treatment
- Provides information about the appropriate increase in treatment in the case of the patient deteriorating
- Provides information about when to seek an urgent medical consultation.

As part of disease-specific education, written action plans have led to significant reductions in hospitalisations (Gibson *et al.* 2010). The evidence for the effectiveness of these action plans was seen across a range of LTCs, from asthma, coronary heart disease and COPD to diabetes (Gibson *et al.* 2010, Murphy *et al.* 2009, Naik *et al.* 2011).

These action plans should be specific to the patient. Each one will be different but they often have the same basic format. This can include:
- Patient identification factors
- Emergency contacts
- List of present medication
- What to do in case…

Look at the reader activity below and consider what you would expect to find listed as the key components in an action plan.

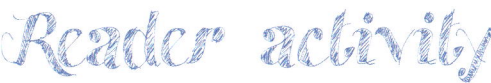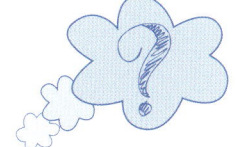

Action plans

- Look at some different action plans (from simple action plans with a traffic light system to a more detailed virtual plan that is stored on iCloud)
- List what components you would include in an action plan you were writing for a particular patient.

Box 11.2: Reader activity – action plans

The House of Care

The House of Care is a model for care of patients with LTCs, which takes into account the expertise and resources of individuals with LTCs and their communities. The aim is to provide a holistic approach to their care and help patients achieve the best possible outcomes (NHS England 2018). The building blocks for high-quality care are the four key interdependent components that are required for person-centred coordinated care. These include:
- Commissioning the appropriate services
- Supporting individuals to self-manage and help them access services
- Organisational and clinical processes that are evidence-based and structured around the needs of patients and carers
- Health and care professionals working in partnership and collaboration.

General Practice Nursing

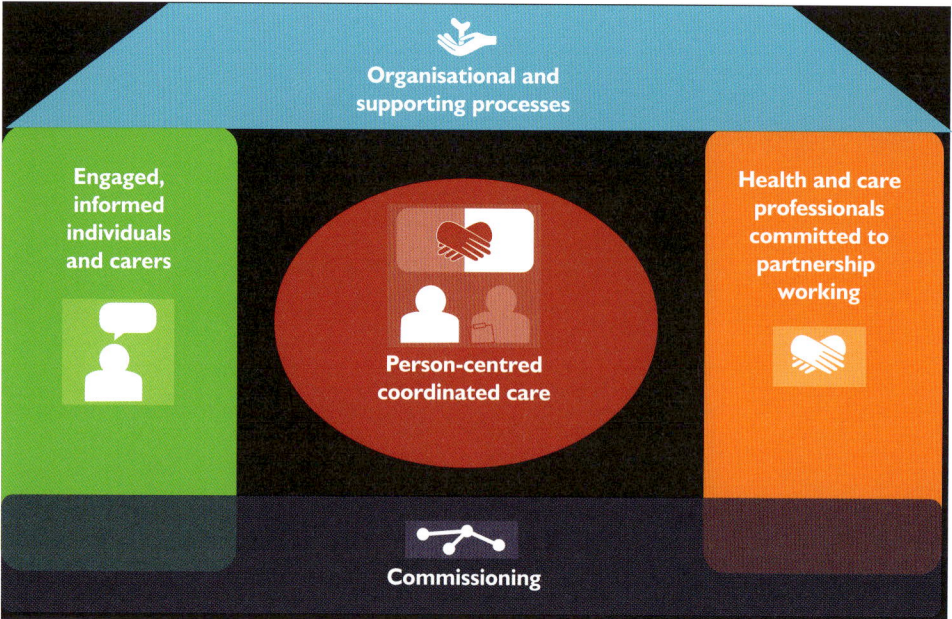

Figure 11.1: House of Care model (NHS England 2018)

Overall there is much emphasis on improving quality of life for people with long-term conditions and their carers. *The Five Year Forward View* (NHS England 2014) stated that, 'long term conditions are now a central task of the NHS; caring for these needs requires a partnership with patients over the longer term rather than providing single, unconnected "episodes" of care.' The aim is to support the rising number of people with long-term conditions, support those with multimorbidity, and help them age well and die well.

Key points from *Liberating the NHS*

- The importance of providing accurate and accessible information to enable people to make informed decisions about their care
- The need for a culture change, to enable patient involvement to become routine in the NHS
- The importance of making 'no decision about me, without me' a reality for everyone, and the concern that, without proper implementation, the proposals might exacerbate health inequalities.

(Adapted from DH 2012b)

Box 11.3: Key points from Liberating the NHS

Mental illness as a long-term condition

There has been a substantial amount of press coverage about mental illness; and there are several mental illnesses that are considered to be long-term conditions, though they have not always been well managed or supported in primary care. One example is long-term depression. There is certainly evidence to show that the management of depression in primary care could be improved. However, there is also a need for substantial investment in primary care services and a major shift in the organisation and provision of care (Gilbody *et al.* 2003). Although there is a chapter later in the book on this topic, we felt it was important to remind the GPN that we care for the whole patient – body, soul and mind.

Summary

As we have seen, a lot of research has been done on long-term conditions. This is partly due to the fact that we have an ageing population and we know the number of patients with LTCs will rise dramatically over the next few years. The research on self-care and self-management shows us that teaching patients to self-manage their care can have a huge impact on their quality of life.

> ### Resources
> **Action plans for asthma:** https://www.asthma.org.uk/advice/manage-your-asthma/action-plan/
>
> **Action plan for diabetes:** https://www.heartfoundation.org.au/after-my-heart-attack/heart-attack-recovery/action-plans/diabetes-action-plan
>
> **National Service Framework for Long-term Conditions:** https://assets.publishing.service.gov.uk/government/uploads/system/uploads/attachment_data/file/198114/National_Service_Framework_for_Long_Term_Conditions.pdf

Box 11:4: Resources

References

Barlow, J., Wright, C., Sheasby, J., Turner, A. & Hainsworth, J. (2002). Self-management approaches for people with chronic conditions: a review. *Patient Education and Counseling.* **48**, 177–87. 10.1016/S0738-3991(02)00032-0.

Barnett, K., Mercer, S.W., Norbury, M., Watt, G., Wyke, S. & Guthrie, B. (2012). Research paper. Epidemiology of multimorbidity and implications for healthcare, research, and medical education: a cross-sectional study. *The Lancet* online. https://www.thelancet.com/pdfs/journals/lancet/PIIS0140-6736%2812%2960240-2.pdf (last accessed 9.4.2019).

Cayton, H. (2006). The flat-pack patient? Creating health together. *Patient Education and Counseling.* **62**, 288–90.

Department of Health (DH) (2012a). *Report. Long-term Conditions Compendium of Information.* 3rd edn https://www.gov.uk/government/news/third-edition-of-long-term-conditions-compendium-published (last accessed 22.1.2019).

Department of Health (DH) (2012b). *Liberating the NHS: No decision about me, without me.* https://assets.publishing.service.gov.uk/government/uploads/system/uploads/attachment_data/file/216980/Liberating-the-NHS-No-decision-about-me-without-me-Government-response.pdf (last accessed 22.1.2019).

Gibson, P.G., Powell, H., Wilson, A., *et al.* (2010). Self-management education and regular practitioner review for adults with asthma [Systematic Review]. Cochrane Database of Systematic Reviews.

Gilbody, S., Whitty, P., Grimshaw, J. & Thomas, R. (2003). Educational and organizational interventions to improve the management of depression in primary care: a systematic review. *Journal of the American Medical Association.* **289**(23), 3145–51.

Kennedy, A., Reeves, D., Bower, P., Lee, V., Middleton, E., Richardson, G., *et al.* (2007). The effectiveness and cost effectiveness of a national lay-led self-care support programme for patients with long-term conditions: a pragmatic randomised controlled trial. *Journal of Epidemiological Community Health.* **61**, 254–61.

Kennedy, A., Bower, P., Reeves, D., Blakeman, T., Bowen, R., Chew-Graham, C., *et al.* (2013). Implementation of self-management support for long term conditions in routine primary care settings: cluster randomised controlled trial. *British Medical Journal.* **346**, f2882.

King's Fund (2011). *Improving the quality of care in general practice: Report of an independent inquiry commissioned by The King's Fund.* https://www.kingsfund.org.uk/publications/improving-quality-care-general-practice (last accessed 22.1.2019).

King's Fund (2018). *Long-term conditions and multi-morbidity.* https://www.kingsfund.org.uk/projects/time-think-differently/trends-disease-and-disability-long-term-conditions-multi-morbidity (last accessed 22.1.2019).

Lorig, K. R., Ritter, P. L., Dost, A., Plant, K., Laurent, D. D. & Mcneil, I. (2008). The Expert Patients Programme online, a 1-year study of an Internet-based self-management programme for people with long-term conditions. *Chronic Illness.* **4**(4), 247–56.

Murphy, A.W., Cupples, M.E., Smith, S.M., Byrne, M., Byrne, M.C. & Newell J. (2009). Effect of tailored practice and patient care plans on secondary prevention of heart disease in general practice: cluster randomised controlled trial. *British Medical Journal.* **339**, b4220

Naik, A.D. *et al.* (2011). Comparative effectiveness of goal setting in diabetes mellitus group clinics: randomized clinical trial. *Archives of Internal Medicine.* **171**, 453–59.

NHS England (2014). *Five year forward view.* https://www.england.nhs.uk/wp-content/uploads/2014/10/5yfv-web.pdf (last accessed 22.1.2019).

NHS England (2018). *House of Care – a framework for long term condition care.* https://www.england.

nhs.uk/ourwork/ltc-op-eolc/ltc-eolc/house-of-care/ (last accessed 22.1.2019).

Parsons, S., Bury, M., Carter, S., Hurst, P., Magee, H. & Taylor, D. (2010). *Self-Management Support amongst Older Adults: The Availability, Impact and Potential of Locally Based Services and Resources. Report for the National Institute for Health Research Service Delivery and Organisation Programme.* London: HMSO.

Ryan, A., Wilson, S., Taylor, A. & Greenfield, S. (2008). Factors associated with self-care activities among adults in the United Kingdom: a systematic review. *BMC Public Health*. **9**, 96.

Taylor, S., Pinnock, H., Epiphaniou, E., Pearce, G., Parke, H., Schwappach, A., Purushotham, J.S., Griffiths, C., Greenhalgh, T. & Sheikh, A. (2014). A rapid synthesis of the evidence on interventions supporting self-management for people with long-term conditions: PRISMS – Practical systematic review of self-management support for long-term conditions. *Health Services and Delivery Research*. No. 2.53

Williams, A.M., Dennis, S. & Harris M.F. (2011). How effective are the linkages between self-management programmes and primary care providers, especially for disadvantaged patients? *Chronic Illness*. **7**, 20–30.

Chapter 12

Diabetes

Sian Hayes

Introduction

In 2016, 3.8 million people over the age of 16 were diagnosed with diabetes – a prevalence rate of 9 per cent of the adult population (PHE 2016). We also know that 90 per cent of adults currently diagnosed with diabetes have type 2 diabetes, which can be prevented or managed by lifestyle changes. In addition, the new Diabetes Prevalence Model, produced by Public Health England and National Cardiovascular Intelligence Network (NCVIN), suggests that 1 in 4 people (25 per cent) with diabetes, an estimated 940,000, are unaware of their condition. This disease can lead to serious complications including foot amputation and kidney disease and is associated with an increased risk of stroke and heart attack.

The proportion of people who have diabetes increases with age: 9 per cent of people aged 45 to 54 have diabetes, but for the over-75s it rises to 23.8 per cent. Diabetes in the elderly has even bigger health implications, as people are more likely to be suffering from other health problems as well, particularly cardiovascular diseases. Diabetes is also increasingly being diagnosed in children. It is more common in men (9.6 per cent, compared with 7.6 per cent in women); and people from South Asian and black ethnic groups are nearly twice as likely to have the disease, compared with people from white, mixed or other ethnic groups (15.2 per cent, compared to 8.0 per cent). Based on current population trends, 4.9 million people will have diabetes by 2035. Type 2 diabetes currently costs the NHS £8.8 billion each year and tackling the rise in the disease is vital to the sustainable future of our healthcare services. The prevalence of diabetes within individual countries in the UK has been recorded by Diabetes UK (2017a).

We therefore diagnose and manage diabetes in order to:

- Relieve its symptoms and reduce the risk of complications
- Prevent death from hyperglycaemic emergencies – diabetic ketoacidosis (DKA) and hyperosmolar hyperglycaemic state (HHS)
- Prevent death from the long-term complications of diabetes.

Table 12.1: WHO recommendations diagnostic criteria for diabetes (WHO 2006)

Diabetes	Fasting plasma glucose 2–h plasma glucose	≥7.0mmol/l (126mg/dl) or ≥11.1mmol/l (200mg/dl)
Impaired glucose tolerance (IGT)	Fasting plasma glucose 2–h plasma glucose	<7.0mmol/l (126mg/dl) and ≥7.8 and <11.1mmol/l (140mg/dl and 200mg/dl)
Impaired fasting glucose (IFG)	Fasting plasma glucose 2–h plasma glucose	6.1 to 6.9mmol/l (110mg/dl to 125mg/dl) and (if measured) <7.8mmol/l (140mg/dl)

Case study: Mrs Smith

We will be following the case of Mrs Smith throughout this chapter (see Box 12.1).

> *Reader activity*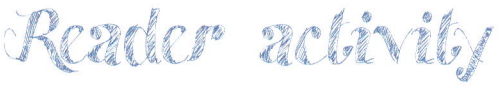
>
> Mrs Smith is 57 years old. She attends the surgery because she is complaining of feeling tired all the time.
>
> Questions to consider:
>
> 1. What do you need to know to make a differential diagnosis?
> 2. What do you think could be her list of differentials?

Box 12.1: Reader activity – case study 1

From the initial conversation, you discover that Mrs Smith's presenting history and clinical symptoms are:
- Slight altered vision
- Feeling thirsty, polyuria (especially nocturia)
- Feeling more tired than usual
- Experiencing episodes of thrush – she normally buys cream over the counter and it clears up.

Additional medical history is as follows:
- Family history – her mum was a type 2 diabetic, diagnosed at the age of 67; father has no relevant history
- Medical history – she missed her health check, as she does not like to attend the surgery unless she has to.

Additional social history is as follows:
- She is normally fit and well, with no relevant past medical history (PMH). She has been trying to lose weight, as she realises her weight has increased in the last few years. She also works full-time in an office. Mrs Smith is married with two older children. She likes to socialise with her husband and friends at weekends.
- Smoking history: She is a social smoker. She tends to smoke when she has a drink at night, between 7 and 10 cigarettes per week.
- Alcohol – she tends to drink wine, approximately 10 units a week (1 unit per night and then approximately 2 units at the weekend).
- Exercise – she does yoga once a week.

Reader activity

Reader activity: Case study 2
Diagnostic tests:
Based on Mrs Smith's history, which initial diagnostic tests do you think need to be done to help you arrive at a diagnosis?
Which tests would you order, from the following list?

continued on next page

> *continued*
> - Fasting glucose
> - U&Es (urea and electrolytes)
> - LFTs (liver function tests)
> - HbA1c
> - Hb
> - ACR (albumin to creatinine ratio)
> - Cholesterol
> - BP (blood pressure)
> - BMI (body mass index)

Box 12.2: Reader activity – case study 2

Diagnosing type 2 diabetes

Table 12.2 is a helpful guide to recognising the symptoms a diabetic patient may present with. Further information is available at WHO (2006).

Table 12.2: Diagnosing type 2 diabetes

SYMPTOMATIC (e.g. polyuria, polydipsia, unexplained weight loss)	ASYMPTOMATIC (According to National guidelines in the UK we would also order two tests for symptomatic people)
A single fasting plasma glucose ≥ 7 or A single random plasma glucose ≥ 11.1	A fasting glucose ≥11.1 on two separate occasions or An HbA1c ≥ 6.5 per cent (48mmol/mol) on two separate occasions two weeks apart or An HbA1c ≥ 6.5 per cent AND a single elevated plasma glucose (fasting ≥ or random ≥11.1) or A random glucose ≥ 11.1 on two separate occasions

HbA1c

HbA1c is the main test for the diagnosis of diabetes

Do not use HbA1c:

- To diagnose type 1 diabetes or in other situations where there is a rapid rise in blood sugar levels (e.g. acute illness, or use of drugs that raise blood sugar rapidly such as oral steroids and antipsychotics)
- If there is increased red cell turnover (including in pregnancy), anaemia and haemoglobinopathies

Please note: this is not a perfect test as an HbA1c of 6.5 per cent/48mmol/mol does not exclude type 2 diabetes.

Mrs Smith had a fasting glucose of 9.4mmol and her HbA1c was 72mmol/mol.

Additional tests

The following tests were also carried out in Mrs Smith's case, to perform a more through health check. The results were:

- Cholesterol: TC 5.8 ratio 5.2
- TFTs, U&Es and LFTs within normal limits
- Anaemia: within normal limits
- Urine: +leucocytes, glucose ++
- BP: 156/90mmHg
- BMI: 40

Mrs Smith was diagnosed with the following problems:

Type 2 diabetes, hypertension and hyperlipidaemia.

It is therefore important to consider the diagnosis of diabetes if patients have the following tell-tale symptoms:

- Increased micturition, especially nocturia
- Polydipsia
- Feeling more tired than usual
- Gaining weight or losing weight without trying to
- Genital itching or thrush
- Cuts and wounds taking longer to heal
- Blurred vision.

Prevention rather than cure

To help tackle the problem, the *Healthier You: NHS Diabetes Prevention Programme* (ICS Health and Wellbeing 2016) was launched by PHE, NHS England and Diabetes UK. The programme is available to those at high risk of type 2 diabetes. It aims to reduce their risk of developing the condition by offering them a referral to an improved diet, weight loss and increased physical activity programme. The NHS DPP will have full coverage across England by 2020. By then, up to 100,000 people will have access to its services each year. People are offered a referral onto the programme through two routes: either through an NHS Health Check appointment (which is offered to men and women aged 40 to 74 who have no other existing cardiovascular health issues), or through identification from GP records. There has been huge enthusiasm from primary care services, with over 185,000 people referred and over 78,000 taking up the programme to date (NHS England April 2018). A digital pathway of the NHS DPP was launched in November 2017.

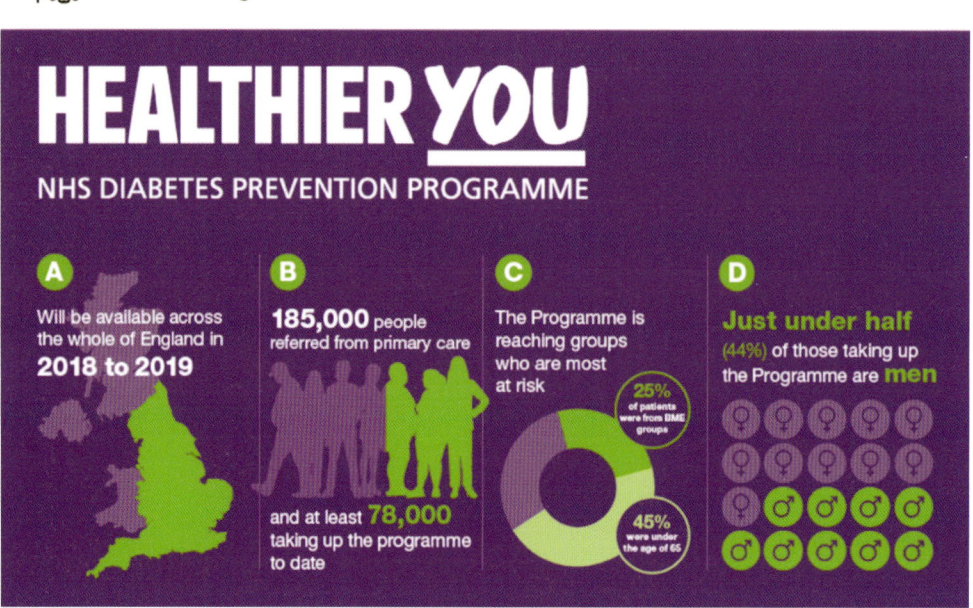

Figure 12.1: Healthier you

There are equivalent programmes in Wales (Health in Wales 2019), Scotland (Scottish Government 2018) and Ireland (Diabetes Ireland 2019).

Diabetes risk factors

The risk factors for diabetes are varied, including:
- Increasing age
- Increasing BMI
- Sedentary lifestyle
- Family history of type 2 diabetes (especially first-degree relatives)
- Ethnicity – South Asian, African, Afro-Caribbean, Chinese
- Gestational diabetes
- Polycystic ovarian syndrome
- Medication, such as corticosteroids and antipsychotics.

You can calculate your own risk score using a self-assessment tool from the Diabetes UK website (Diabetes UK 2019).

Managing diabetes
Mrs Smith's treatment plan

Mrs Smith was initially started on metformin 500mg once a day, then increased up to 4 a day (two tablets, twice a day). This is in line with the NICE guidelines (2017). The main side effect of this medicine is gastrointestinal upset. It is therefore advised that metformin is taken with food. For further side effects, check the current British National Formulary online (BNF Publications 2019).

Metformin is typically the first-line drug treatment (Davies *et al.* 2018) but titration is essential:

- Begin with low-dose metformin (500mg), taken once per day with meals (breakfast or dinner). Advise the patient that they may experience some gastrointestinal (GI) side effects to start with, and that it is important to take the medication with food to reduce this risk.
- After 7 days, if GI side effects have settled, advance the dose to 500 mg twice per day (medication to be taken before breakfast and dinner).
- Increase by 500mg each week until the maximum effective dose is reached. This is usually 2g daily in divided doses. A diabetes specialist may increase it to 3g if tolerated.
- GI side effects may appear as the dose is increased. If these do not settle, decrease to previous lower dose and try to increase the dose again at a later time.

- Metformin modified release (MR) tablets can be tried in patients who cannot tolerate the standard release tablets.
- Combination products including metformin can improve compliance and concordance, but they can also make it more difficult to carry out titration.

The other management issues that should be discussed are:
- Patient education and lifestyle modification – individualised care plans
- Monitoring to prevent and detect early complications
- Glycaemic control, looking for both hyperglycaemia and hypoglycaemia
- Cardiovascular risk reduction
- Referral for eye screening
- Ensuring that we don't make living with diabetes intolerable through intrusive drug regimes, monitoring or expectations.

(NICE 2016).

Which needs lowering most urgently, blood sugar, cholesterol or BP?

For people with diabetes, controlling blood pressure and cholesterol is even more important than blood sugar control in order to reduce the risk of macrovascular complications such as heart attacks or stroke. The recommended guidelines for blood sugar, cholesterol and BP are summarised in an American study (ACC/AHA 2013). Poor glucose control is associated with increased mortality and an increased risk of microvascular complications so it is also very important.

Patient education and lifestyle modification

Being obese is the main modifiable risk factor for type 2 diabetes (PHE 2014). In fact, obese adults in England are five times more likely to be diagnosed with diabetes than adults of a healthy weight (PHE 2014). Education and lifestyle modification are therefore vital aspects of the GPN's role when caring for patients with diabetes.

Dietary advice

There is no specific recommended diet. However, there is evidence that the 'Mediterranean' eating pattern reduced HbA1c more than control diets. Low-carbohydrate, low glycaemic index and high-protein diets and the dietary approach to stop hypertension (DASH) diet have all improved glycaemic control (Esposito *et al.* 2015).

For dietary advice, the best course of action is to refer patients to the dietician and education courses that support lifestyle education such as DESMOND (2018). People with type 2 diabetes should be offered access to ongoing diabetes self-management education and support via the DSMES Toolkit (CDC 2018). DSMES can promote medication adherence, healthy eating and physical activity. It is cost-effective and can improve outcomes and glycaemic control and reduce hospital admissions and all-cause mortality.

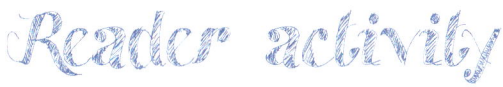

Diabetes education

Find out about your local educational provision for lifestyle advice for patients with both type 1 and type 2 diabetes.

Box 12.3: Reader activity – diabetes education

Weight loss measures

Check whether the patient's BMI is over 25 and take their waist measurement, as this is an indicator of central obesity – visceral fat makes people insulin-resistant. If their BMI is greater than 35, and if patients are willing and motivated, and after other options have failed, they will be offered bariatric surgery. This has been NHS policy since 2013 (NICE 2013).

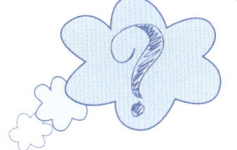

Bariatric surgery

Find out what your local policy is on bariatric surgery and whether any patients in your surgery have had bariatric surgery.

Box 12.4: Reader activity – bariatric surgery

Case study continued

Six months later Mrs Smith attended the surgery. She had some more tests done and these were the results:

- HbA1c – 62mmol/mol
- BP – 150/86mmHg,
- Cholesterol – TC 5.2 ratio 4.8
- BMI – 39
- ACR <2

Mrs Smith had tried to alter her eating habits and lose weight by cutting out cakes and biscuits at work, and eating sensibly with fewer carbohydrates and more vegetables. She had also tried to go to the gym but hurt her back so she stopped while it improved but has been walking frequently. Consider the patient factors in Box 12.5 (below).

Specific factors that affect choice of treatment
- Individualised HbA1c target
- Impact on weight and hypoglycaemia
- Side effect profile of medication
- Complexity of regimen (frequency of dose, mode of administration, etc.)
- Regimen to optimise adherence and persistence
- Access, cost and availability of medication

Patient characteristics
- Current lifestyle
- Comorbidities (e.g. atherosclerotic cardiovascular disease [ASCVD], renal disease or chronic kidney disease [CKD] and heart failure [HF])
- Clinical characteristics – age, HbA1c, weight
- Issues of motivation and depression
- Cultural and socioeconomic context

Box 12.5: Patient factors

Further treatment options

There are a few treatment options that can be considered. These include:
- Another non insulin blood glucose lowering therapy in combination (dual therapy), e.g. metformin and DPP-4 (gliptins), SGL2i (NICE 2017).

- An angiotensin converting enzyme inhibitor (ACEi) such as Lisinopril to provide renal protection.
- A statin for cholesterol lowering activity. Once good control has been established, NICE (2017) advises that HbA1c should be rechecked every 6 months, not just at annual review. If control has not been met, then treatment should be assessed and modified 3–6 monthly to avoid clinical inertia (failure to intensify therapy when treatment targets are not met). Having a multidisciplinary team that includes specialist nurses or pharmacists may help reduce inertia as well as a coordinated chronic care model. Consideration must be given to any underlying cause, e.g. excess weight or renal impairment.

ADULT WITH TYPE 2 DIABETES WHO CAN TAKE METFORMIN

If HbA1c rises to 48mmol/mol (6.5%) on lifestyle interventions:
- Offer standard-release metformin
- Support the person to aim for an HbA1c level of 48mmol/mol (6.5%)

If standard release metformin is not tolerated, consider a trial of modified-release metformin

FIRST INTENSIFICATION
If HbA1c rises to 58mmol/mol (7.5%):
- Consider dual therapy with:
  - metformin and a DPP-4i
  - metformin and pioglitazone
  - metformin and an SU
  - *metformin and an SGLT-2i*
- Support the person to aim for an HbA1c level of 53mmol/mol (7.0%)

SECOND INTENSIFICATION
If HbA1c rises to 58mmol/mol (7.5%):
- Consider triple therapy with:
  - metformin, a DPP-4i and an SU
  - metformin, pioglitazone and an SU
  - *metformin, pioglitazone and an SU and an SGLT-2i*
  - insulin based treatment
- Support the person to aim for an HbA1c level of 53mmol/mol (7.0%)

If triple therapy is not effective, not tolerated or contraindicated, consider combination therapy with metformin, an SU and a GLP-1 mimetic for adults with type 2 diabetes who:
- *have a BMI of 35kg/m² or higher (adjust accordingly for people from black, Asian and other minority ethnic groups) and specific psychological or other medical problems associated with obesity or*
- *have a BMI lower than 35kg/m², and for whom insulin therapy would have significant occupational implications, or weight loss would benefit other obesity related comorbidities.*

Box 12.6: NICE (2017) diabetes management recommendations

Home blood glucose monitoring (HBGM)
NICE (2017) recommends that patients should not routinely be offered blood glucose monitoring unless:
- They are on insulin treatment
- There is evidence that they are experiencing hypoglycaemic episodes
- They are on oral medication that may increase their risk of hypoglycaemia while driving or operating machinery
- They are pregnant or planning to become pregnant

Discuss the *At a Glance Guide to the Current Medical Standards of Fitness to Drive* (DVLA 2012)

The Diabetes UK literature on Meds and Kit explains all the different monitors (Diabetes UK 2017b). You need to familiarise yourself with the ones used in your practice.

Cholesterol
Primary prevention is to reduce non-HDL cholesterol to 40 per cent (NICE 2014). The medication of choice is atorvastatin or, if this is not tolerated, other statins. If total cholesterol is around 5.3 and LDL 3.8, offer atorvastatin 40mg. For secondary prevention (such as post-MI), the recommended medication is atorvastatin 80mg.

Note:
- Statins may increase proteinuria at first so it's advisable to wait 1 month, then repeat blood tests.
- This treatment can also cause hypothyroidism (McFadden *et al.* 2014).

• Blood pressure
The aim of good blood pressure control is to set a target blood pressure of <130/80mmHg for people with kidney, eye or cardiovascular damage. For others, set a target blood pressure <140/80 mmHg (NICE 2017).

Diabetes

> ### Reader activity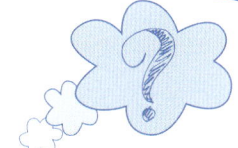
>
> Mrs Smith needs to have a pre-review of her diabetes before her annual review.
>
> Which of the following tests should be considered?
> - HbA1c
> - Cholesterol
> - LFT
> - U&Es
> - GFR
> - B12
> - TFT
> - Urine sample for ACR
> - BP
> - Waist measurement

Box 12.7: Reader activity – further review

The results of Mrs Smith's annual review are as follows:

- HbA1c – 76mmol/mol
- Cholesterol – TC 4.2, HDL 1.78 ratio 3.2
- The blood tests B12, TFT, LFT, U&Es and GFR were all within normal limits
- Her ACR was <2
- Her blood pressure reading was 138/78mmHg
- Her waist measurement was 94cm.
- Foot check – pulses within normal limits. Her sensation was good with normal vibration.

Additional information:

She mentioned that, due to her back problem, she has not exercised as much as she would have liked. Her weight has increased. She is also experiencing a low mood due

to her condition. Mrs Smith informed the GPN that she has not had any side effects from the medication. The following is a list of her prescribed medication:
- Dual therapy (metformin and alogliptin)
- Lisinopril 5mg
- Atorvastatin 10mg

Case study (continued)

The role of the GPN is to help Mrs Smith reach her targets with her weight, blood pressure and control of her HbA1c. There will therefore need to be a discussion about diet, exercise and other lifestyle choices. The new treatment approach by ADA/EASD (2018) takes into consideration the benefits of some of the drugs – specific SGLT2i and GLP-1 reduce mortality, heart failure and progression of renal disease.

However, prescribers need to consider a history of atherosclerotic CVD (ASCVD), HF and CKD, very early in the process of deciding on treatment options. These conditions are known to affect 15–20 per cent of the population with type 2 diabetes (ADA/EASD 2018). DPP-4 inhibitors have demonstrated cardiovascular safety but not benefits and both alogliptin and saxagliptin are subject to FDA warnings against use in heart failure.

In some cases, triple therapy may be preferable. This involves taking another tablet, GLP1 or insulin or changing alogliptin to an SGLT2 inhibitor. SGLT2 inhibitors cause their glucose- lowering effect in an insulin-dependent manner by reducing renal glucose reabsorption, leading to increased excretion of glucose in the urine. Around 300kcal glucose is excreted daily so, in addition to improvements in glycaemic control, this class of drug can also lead to weight loss.

In May 2017, NICE revised their 2015 treatment guideline, placing great emphasis on the use of SGLT2 inhibitors as second-line therapy options, alongside gliptins, pioglitazone and sulphonylureas (SUs). They also advocate the use of SGLT2i in triple therapy (NICE 2017). GPNs will therefore need to check with their practice whether they are able to prescribe, or whether you need a diabetic consultant authority to prescribe. They will also need to give the patient information on diabetic ketoacidosis (DKA). One leaflet has been developed by Diabetes UK TREND (TREND 2016). Patients with established CVD appear to have cardiovascular benefit with some SGLT2 inhibitors (ADA/EASD 2018).

In Mrs Smith's case, you can also consider a GLP-1 receptor agonist (glucagon-like peptide-1), as her BMI is above 35. An assessment of the patient's cardiovascular risk is required, as some GLP-1s (such as liraglutide) have stronger evidence for CVD benefit. In some areas you need to sign a contract with the surgery, as you can only continue GLP1 mimetic therapy if the person has a beneficial metabolic response – a reduction of HbA1c by at least 11mmol/mol (1 per cent) and a weight loss of at least 3 per cent of initial body weight in 6 months.

Full efforts to achieve glycaemic and blood pressure targets and to follow guidelines for lipid management, antiplatelet and antithrombotic therapy and smoking cessation should also be priorities in managing type 2 diabetes.

Patients generally need a mood assessment, with referral to their GP if their mood remains low. It might also be appropriate to refer them to another local GPN who specialises in insulin initiation (either in the surgery or with a Diabetes Specialist Nurse). There may also be a referral to secondary care for further education, if insulin is decided on.

In Mrs Smith's case, she wanted to try the SGLT2i instead of the alogliptin. The GPN discussed portion sizes and an altered diet. The GPN also discussed Mrs Smith's ability to increase exercise and she was offered a GP exercise referral. She also continued her statins and ACE inhibitors.

> *Reader activity*
>
> **Exercise referral**
>
> Find out what your local exercise referral programme is and see what the uptake is in your area.

Box 12.8. Reader activity – exercise referral

Mrs Smith was started on SGLT2i (empagliflozin) 25mg, with her metformin. The alogliptin was stopped as she didn't consider it effective. Side effects were discussed and she was given the information sheet on sick day rules and DKA and is due to be seen in 3 months' time for another blood test and review of symptoms.

Key recommendations

- Offer ongoing diabetes self-management education and support (DSMES) to all patients with type 2 diabetes (T2D)
- Consider medication adherence when selecting glucose-lowering medications
- For patients with T2D and CVD, offer an SGLT2i or GLP-IRA with proven cardiovascular benefit
- For patients with ASCVD and HF, offer an SGLT2i
- For patients with T2D and CKD, consider an SGLT2i (or GLP-IRA) with renal benefits
- All overweight and obese patients should be encouraged to engage in an intensive lifestyle management programme that may include food substitution
- Encourage participation in increased physical activity, which improves glycaemic control. To avoid clinical inertia, reassess and modify treatment regularly (at 3- to 6-monthly intervals).

(Davies et al. 2018)

Box 12.9: Key recommendations

It is important to note that tissue damage is preventable if patients are supported to:
- Keep blood glucose near normal
- Keep blood pressure normal
- Reduce other cardiovascular risk factors, e.g. smoking, obesity and hyperlipidaemia
- Carry out self-care by monitoring their blood glucose levels, diet and exercise, and attend regular screening and health checks
- Recognise tissue damage early – and get appropriate referral, e.g. for podiatry.

Complications of diabetes

The complications are diabetes are related to hyperglycaemia. They can be separated into macrovascular complications (coronary artery disease, peripheral arterial disease and stroke) and microvascular complications (diabetic nephropathy, neuropathy, and retinopathy) (Diabetes UK 2019b).

Macrovascular complications of diabetes

The central pathological mechanism in macrovascular disease is the process of atherosclerosis, which leads to the narrowing of arterial walls throughout the body. Atherosclerosis is thought to result from chronic inflammation and injury to the arterial wall in the peripheral or coronary vascular system. In response to endothelial injury and inflammation, oxidised lipids from low-density lipoprotein (LDL) particles accumulate in the endothelial wall of arteries.

Monocytes infiltrate the vessel wall and convert into macrophages, which accumulate oxidised lipids to form foam cells. The foam cells stimulate macrophage proliferation and attraction of T-lymphocytes. T-lymphocytes, in turn, induce smooth muscle proliferation in the blood vessel wall and collagen accumulation. The result is the formation of a lipid-rich atherosclerotic lesion with a fibrous cap. Rupture of this lesion leads to acute vascular infarction. In addition to atheroma formation, there is strong evidence of increased platelet adhesion and hypercoagulability in type 2 diabetes. The resulting complications can therefore be coronary artery disease, peripheral arterial disease and stroke.

Microvascular disease

Microvascular disease affects the finer blood vessels in the body, which include the capillaries. There is a thickening of the basement membrane of capillaries, causing leakage or blockage of the transfer of nutrients and waste substances. It is also associated with retinopathy, nephropathy and neuropathy.

Diabetic retinopathy

Diabetic retinopathy is the most common form of microvascular complication of diabetes (NICE 2017). Diabetic retinopathy is defined as 'a chronic progressive, potentially sight-threatening disease of the retinal microvasculature associated with the prolonged hyperglycaemia and other conditions linked to diabetes mellitus such as hypertension' (Royal College of Ophthalmologists 2014). The risk of developing diabetic retinopathy is known to increase with age, as well as with less well controlled blood sugar and blood pressure levels.

According to the NHS, 1,280 new cases of blindness caused by diabetic retinopathy are reported each year in England alone, while a further 4,200 people in the country are thought to be at risk of retinopathy-related vision loss (Diabetes UK 2017a). Interestingly, although the incidence of diabetes is increasing, that of diabetic retinopathy is falling. This is probably largely due to better management of glucose levels, lipid abnormalities and hypertension (Antonetti *et al.* 2012).

Diabetic nephropathy

Diabetic nephropathy is the leading cause of renal failure, so every person with diabetes type 1 or 2 should be tested for CKD using eGFR, creatinine and ACR (NICE 2018). This condition is defined by proteinuria >500mg in 24 hours in the setting of diabetes, and this is preceded by lower degrees of proteinuria, or 'microalbuminuria'. Microalbuminuria is defined as albumin excretion of 30–299mg per 24 hours (NICE 2017). The damage to the kidney includes increased glomerular basement membrane thickness, microaneurysm formation and mesangial nodule formation.

The initial priority is prevention, as there are strong associations between controlling glucose and reducing the risk of developing diabetic nephropathy. Patients should be treated to the lowest safe glucose level that can be obtained to prevent or control diabetic nephropathy. This is also true of hypertension, as tight control of blood pressure will lead to a decline in glomerular filtration rate (GFR).

Diabetic neuropathy

Diabetic neuropathy affects all the peripheral nerves, including sensory neurons and motor neurons, but rarely affects the autonomic nervous system. A patient can have sensorimotor and autonomic neuropathy or any other combination. Signs and symptoms vary depending on the nerve or nerves affected (Fowler 2008). It has been suggested that more than 80 per cent of amputations occur after foot ulceration or injury due to diabetic neuropathy (Boulton *et al.* 2005); see also the diabetic.co.uk website (2018) for these conditions.

Long-term effects of microvascular disease

The long-term effects include:

- Retinopathy – blindness
- Nephropathy – renal failure
- Neuropathy – amputation
- Erectile dysfunction – sexual dysfunction is complex and often leads to poor self-image, embarrassment and guilt. Men with type 2 diabetes should be given the opportunity to discuss erectile dysfunction as part of their annual review (NICE 2017). Phosphodiesterase 5 inhibitors can be prescribed to treat problematic erectile dysfunction (NICE 2017).
- Charcot joints – Charcot foot is a condition causing weakening of the bones in the foot that can occur in people who have significant nerve damage (neuropathy). The bones are weakened enough to fracture and, with continued walking, the foot eventually changes shape. Certainly, patients who have a foot deformity due to Charcot arthropathy are at high risk of ulceration and should be cared for by the foot protection service (NICE 2016).

Annual screening

The diabetic eye screening programme in England aims to invite all people with diabetes, aged 12 or over, for retinal photography to screen for the presence of diabetic retinopathy (Harris 2012). Various tests are also carried out annually to identify and monitor these conditions.

Microalbuminuria is asymptomatic so annual screening is required – using the urinary albumin to creatinine ratio (ACR). A first-pass urine sample is preferable, as it gives a more accurate result. In case of false positives, heavy exercise and urinary tract infection (UTI), repeat the ACR. A normal result is <3mg/mmol. If the ACR is raised, patients are advised to reduce their BP to 135/75mmHg. Raised BP should be treated with ACE inhibitors, as they are cardioprotective and renoprotective.

Insulin

This is a huge topic but these are the main aspects to consider in insulin therapy. It's best to start by finding out which types of insulin are used in your practice. Familiarise yourself with the types and why they are used. You should also refer to the Diabetic Specialist Team, the diabetes.org.uk website and NICE guidelines (2017) to assist you in administering insulin therapy.

Some key points to remember are as follows:
- Replace the background (basal) insulin, e.g. Insulatard, Humulin I, Levemir, Lantus
- Or replace the mealtime (bolus) insulin, e.g. Novorapid, Apidra, Humalog
- Or replace both, e.g. Humulin M3, Novomix 30, Humalog mix 25 and 50.

The diabetes.org.uk website has a really good pamphlet on insulin and the pens it's delivered in – called Meds and Kits (Diabetes UK 2017b).

Insulin therapy for type 2 diabetics

If you sit in with a Diabetic Specialist Nurse, you will find a great deal of information that needs to be covered when starting a patient on insulin:
- Insulin therapy – first-line NPH insulin, i.e. Humulin I or Insuman basal
- Normally the patient is started on insulin based on their body weight – e.g. 10 per cent body weight of 80kg would be 8 units. The dose is then increased by 2 units every 2–3 days until Fasting Blood Sugar (FBS) is around 7–8mmol – patient responsibility (normally given once a day, 30 minutes before evening meal or bed)
- Important points to discuss:
  - Blood monitoring using a hand-held device before and after meal.
  - Injection technique – how, when and where (FIT recommendations)

- Lipohypertrophy
- Hypoglycaemia and management, hyperglycaemia
- Storage of insulin
- Safe disposal of needles – sharps
- Driving
- Insurance
- Sick day rules
- Contacts if concerned
- Direct patient to diabetes.org.uk, where they can sign up to get support
- Referral to education programme for insulin initiation for the patient
- What are the possible emergencies that may arise for a person with diabetes?
- Managing any emergencies – what do you know regarding:
  - Diabetic ketoacidosis (DKA)
  - Hyperosmolar hyperglycaemic state (HHS)
  - Hypoglycaemia?

Diabetic ketoacidosis (DKA)

This mainly occurs in patients with type 1 diabetes, but anyone on insulin or on SGLT2i could develop it. DKA is a serious problem condition caused by the body running out of insulin. Insulin is needed to allow glucose to enter the cells for energy. In its absence, the body breaks down fat as a source of energy, and ketones build up.

The times when it is most likely to occur are:
- At diagnosis, when patients are ill
- During a growth spurt or puberty
- When patients have not taken insulin for any reason
- DKA usually develops over 24 hours but can develop faster, particularly in young children. Hospital admission and treatment is essential to correct the life-threatening acidosis. Treatment tends to involve monitoring, and administration of IV fluids, insulin and glucose.

DKA can also be accompanied by high blood glucose levels – above 15mmol.

Signs and symptoms include:
- Frequently passing urine, thirst, feeling tired and lethargic, blurry vision
- Abdominal pain, nausea, vomiting, breathing changes (deep sighing breaths)
- Smell of ketones on breath (often likened to smell of pear drops), collapsing/unconsciousness.

Anybody who is on insulin or SGL2 should be monitored for ketones if their blood glucose is over 15mmol/l (NICE 2017).

Advise patients as follows:
- Always take diabetes medication particularly insulin, even if they feel unwell and can't eat but omit metformin if not eating due to lactic acidosis (sick day rules)
- Test blood sugars more frequently
- Contact the healthcare team if concerned – and blood glucose levels remain high (>15mmol/l)
- Drink plenty of unsweetened fluids
- If they can't eat, replace meals with snacks and drinks, containing carbohydrate.

When carrying out a blood ketone test:
- Lower than 0.6mmol/L is a normal reading
- 0.6 to 1.5mmol/L means a slightly increased risk of DKA and they should test again in a couple of hours
- 1.6 to 2.9mmol/L means increased risk of DKA and the patient should contact the Diabetes Team or GP as soon as possible
- 3mmol/L or over means a very high risk of DKA and they need emergency medical help.

(See TREND 2016, 2018)

Hypoglycaemia

The definition of hypoglycaemia is when blood glucose is <4mmol. Patients may have some or all of the following symptoms:
- Sweating
- Fatigue
- Dizziness
- Pallor
- Fatigue
- Feeling hungry
- A raised heart rate
- Blurred vision
- Temporary loss of consciousness
- Confusion
- Convulsions

In extreme cases, patients can go into a coma.

Immediate treatment should be administration of glucose (e.g. 5 jelly babies). The patient will need their blood sugar checked 15 minutes later. If the blood sugar is still low, repeat the process. Please refer to TREND (2013) or other hypo leaflets to provide the patient with all the information required.

Hyperosmolar hyperglycaemic state (HHS)

HHS occurs in people with type 2 diabetes who experience very high blood glucose levels (often over 40mmol/l). The body is trying to get rid of the excess sugar. It can develop over several weeks through a combination of illness and dehydration. Stopping diabetes medication during illness can contribute, but blood glucose often rises despite the usual diabetes medication because of other hormones the body produces during illness.

Symptoms frequently include: urination, thirst, nausea, dry skin, disorientation and, in later stages, drowsiness and a gradual loss of consciousness.

The patient should be admitted to hospital to correct dehydration and bring their blood glucose down to an acceptable level by giving replacement fluid and IV insulin. HHS does not usually lead to the presence of ketones in the urine, as occurs in DKA. Because people with type 2 diabetes may still be producing some insulin, ketones may not be created.

Reader activity

Mrs Smith needs to have a review of her diabetes prior to her annual review.
Which of the following tests should be considered?

- HbA1c
- Cholesterol
- LFTs
- U&Es
- GFR
- B12
- TFTs
- Urine sample for ACR
- BP
- Waist measurement

Box 12.10: Reader activity – further review (answers on p. 130)

Summary

GPNs offer diabetes education and yearly reviews, and advise on and, in many cases, prescribe medication. For many type 2 diabetics, the practice nurse is their regular point of contact in general practice and they see their doctor very seldom. The good news is that HbA1c outcomes are the same, whether patients are managed by nurses or GPs.

Key things to note are:

- Adhere to the NICE guidelines for diabetes – see: https://www.nice.org.uk/guidance/conditions-and-diseases/diabetes-and-other-endocrinal--nutritional-and-metabolic-conditions (last accessed 28/01/2019).
- The blood glucose control should be optimised to HbA1c <7.5 per cent 58mmol/mol for prevention of microvascular disease, and ≤6.5 per cent 48mmol/mol for increased arterial risk.
- Cardiovascular risk must be assessed annually using the UK Prospective Diabetes Study risk tool (Stevens *et al.* 2012).
- You also need to consider microalbuminuria, features of metabolic syndrome and conventional risk factors such as familial hypercholesterolaemia, abnormal lipid profile, BP and smoking.

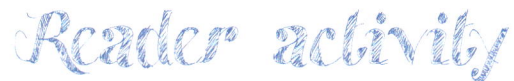

Differential diagnosis

Think about the case of Mrs Smith.

1. What do you need to know to make a differential diagnosis?
    - Do you need to take a more in-depth history?
    - Do you need to carry out additional tests?
2. What do you think could be her list of differentials?
    - Type 2 diabetes
    - Hypothyroidism
    - Anaemia
    - Vitamin D deficiency
    - Urine infection/thrush

Box 12.11: Reader activity – differential diagnosis

Reader activity

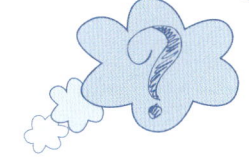

Reader activity box 12.10: Answers

- HbA1c (True)
- Cholesterol (True)
- LFT (True)
- U&Es (True)
- GFR (True)
- B12 (False)
- TFTs (True)
- Urine sample for ACR (True)
- BP (True)
- Waist measurement (False)

Box 12.12: Answers to reader activity – further review

References

American College of Cardiology/American Heart Association (ACC/AHA) (2013). *Guideline on the Treatment of Blood Cholesterol to Reduce Atherosclerotic Cardiovascular Risk in Adults.* https://www.ahajournals.org/doi/full/10.1161/01.cir.0000437738.63853.7a (last accessed 9.2.2019).

American Diabetes Association and the European Association for the Study of Diabetes (ADA/EASD) (2018). *Updated ADA, EASD Consensus Guidelines for Managing Hyperglycemia in T2D.* https://www.endocrinologyadvisor.com/home/topics/diabetes/type-2-diabetes/updated-ada-easd-consensus-guidelines-for-managing-hyperglycemia-in-t2d/

Antonetti, D., Klein, R.R. & Gardner, T.W. (2012). Diabetic retinopathy. *New England Journal of Medicine.* **366**, 1227–39. https://www.nejm.org/doi/full/10.1056/NEJMra1005073 (last accessed 26.1.2019).

Boulton, A.J., Vinik, A.I., Arezzo, J.C., Bril, V., Feldman, E.L., Freeman, R., Malik, R.A., Maser, R.E., Sosenko, J.M. & Ziegler, D. (2005). Diabetic neuropathies: a statement by the American Diabetes Association. *Diabetes Care.* **28**, 956–62.

BNF Publications (2019). https://www.bnf.org/products/bnf-online/ (last accessed 26.1.2019).

Centers for Disease Control and Prevention (CDC) (2018). *DSMES Toolkit.* https://www.cdc.gov/diabetes/dsmes-toolkit/index.html (last accessed 26.1.2019).

Cheyette, C. & Balolia, Y. (2013). *Carbs and Cals.* 5th edn. London: Chello Publishing.

Davies, M.J., D'Alessio, D.A, Fradkin, *et al.* (2018). Management of hyperglycaemia in type 2 diabetes. A consensus report by the American Diabetes Association (ADA) and the European Association for the study of Diabetes (EASD). *Diabetes Care.* **41**(12), 2669–701. doi: 10.2337/dci18-0033.

DESMOND (2018). https://www.desmond-project.org.uk/ (last accessed 26.1.2019).

Diabetes.co.uk (2018). *Diabetic Retinopathy.* http://www.diabetes.co.uk/diabetes-complications/diabetic-retinopathy.html (last accessed 26.1.2019).

Diabetes Ireland (2019). *Eat well to prevent type 2 diabetes.* https://www.diabetes.ie/living-with-diabetes/are-you-at-risk/low-risk/eat-well-prevent-type-2-diabetes/ (last accessed 26.1.2019).

Diabetes UK (2017a). *Diabetes Prevalence 2017.* https://www.diabetes.org.uk/professionals/position-statements-reports/statistics/diabetes-prevalence-2017 (last accessed 26.1.2019).

Diabetes UK (2017b). *Meds & Kit.* https://shop.diabetes.org.uk/products/meds-and-kits (last accessed 26.1.2019).

Diabetes UK (2019a). *Type 2 diabetes: Know your risk.* https://riskscore.diabetes.org.uk/start?_ga=2.160594680.451160947.1548258601-1542326537.1548258601(last accessed 26.1.2019).

Diabetes UK (2019b). https://www.diabetes.org.uk/ (last accessed 26.1.2019).

Driver and Vehicle Licensing Agency (DVLA) (2012). https://bpna.org.uk/pr3ss/wp-content/uploads/2012/04/9.2-DVLA.pdf (last accessed 9.2.2019).

Esposito, K., Maiorino, M.I., Bellastella, G., Chiodini, P., Panagiotakos, D. & Giugliano, D. (2015). A journey into a Mediterranean diet and type 2 diabetes: a systematic review with meta-analyses. *British Medical Journal.* **5**(8). https://bmjopen.bmj.com/content/5/8/e008222 (last accessed 7.2.2019).

Fowler, M. (2008). Microvascular and Macrovascular Complications of Diabetes. *Clinical Diabetes.* **26**(2), 77–82. https://doi.org/10.2337/diaclin.26.2.77 (last accessed 26.1.2019).

Harris, M. (2012). *The NHS Diabetic Eye Screening Programme: New Common Pathway.* The Royal College of Ophthalmologists. London: Focus.

Health in Wales (2019). http://www.wales.nhs.uk/preventingdiabetes (last accessed 26.1.2019).

ICS Health and Wellbeing (2016). *Diabetes prevention.* https://icshealth.co.uk/our-services/diabetes-prevention/ (last accessed 26.1.2019).

McFadden, E., Jones, M.E., Schoemaker, M.J., Ashworth, A. & Swerdlow, A.J. (2014). The relationship between obesity and exposure to light at night: cross-sectional analyses of over 100,000 women in the Breakthrough Generations Study. *American journal of epidemiology,* **180**(3), 245-250.

NHS (2018). *Diabetic eye screening.* https://www.nhs.uk/Conditions/diabetic-eye-screening/ (last accessed 26.1.2019).

NICE (2013). *Obesity: identification, assessment and management.* https://www.nice.org.uk/guidance/cg189/chapter/1-recommendations (last accessed 28.01.2019).

NICE (2016). *Diabetic foot problems: prevention and management. NICE guideline [NG19]* Published date: August 2015. Last updated: January 2016.

NICE (2017). *Type 2 diabetes in adults: management. NICE guideline [NG28]* Published date: December 2017.

NIH (2018). *Diabetic neuropathy.* https://www.niddk.nih.gov/health-information/diabetes/overview/preventing-problems/nerve-damage-diabetic-neuropathies. (last accessed 26.1.2019).

Public Health England (2014). *Adult obesity and type 2 diabetes.* https://assets.publishing.service.gov.uk/government/uploads/system/uploads/attachment_data/file/338934/Adult_obesity_and_type_2_diabetes_.pdf (last accessed 26.1.2019).

Stevens, R.J., Kothari, V., Adler, A.I., Stratton, I.M. & Holman, R.R. on behalf of the United Kingdom Prospective Diabetes Study (UKPDS) Group. (2012). The UKPDS risk engine: a model for the risk of coronary heart disease in Type II diabetes (UKPDS 56). *Clinical Science.* **101**, 671–79. https://www.dtu.ox.ac.uk/riskengine/ukpds56.pdf (last accessed 26.1.2019).

Royal College of Ophthalmologists (2013). *Diabetic Retinopathy Guidelines.* https://www.rcophth.ac.uk/wp-content/uploads/2014/12/2013-SCI-301-FINAL-DR-GUIDELINES-DEC-2012-updated-July-2013.pdf (last accessed 26.1.2019).

Scottish Government (2018). *A Healthier Future: type 2 Diabetes prevention, early detection and intervention: framework.* https://www.gov.scot/publications/healthier-future-framework-prevention-early-detection-early-intervention-type-2/ (last accessed 26.1.2019).

TREND (2013). http://trend-uk.org/wp-content/uploads/2017/02/Hypo-leaflet-V4.pdf (last accessed 26.1.2019).

TREND (2016). *Type 2 diabetes and diabetic ketoacidosis.* http://trend-uk.org/wp-content/uploads/2017/02/TREND-DKA-4pp-patient-leaflet-spreads_screen.pdf (last accessed 26.1.2019).

TREND (2018). *Type 1 diabetes: What to do when you are ill.* http://trend-uk.org/wp-content/uploads/2018/03/A5_T1Illness_TREND_FINAL.pdf (last accessed 26.1.2019).

World Health Organization (WHO) (2006). *Definition and diagnosis of diabetes mellitus and intermediate hyperglycemia.* https://www.who.int/diabetes/publications/Definition%20and%20diagnosis%20of%20diabetes_new.pdf (last accessed 26.1.2019).

Chapter 13

Respiratory conditions

Deborah Duncan

Introduction

The General Practice Nurse will meet patients with a range of respiratory conditions, which can be separated into obstructive and restrictive diseases. This chapter will focus on assessing and managing two of the most common long-term respiratory conditions, asthma and chronic obstructive pulmonary disease (COPD). 'Chronic respiratory diseases are a group of chronic diseases affecting the airways and the other structures of the lungs' (WHO 2007, p. 12). These are asthma, chronic obstructive pulmonary disease, bronchiectasis, hypersensitivity pneumonia, lung fibrosis, chronic pleural diseases, pneumoconiosis, pulmonary eosinophilia, sarcoidosis and sleep apnoea syndrome and cancer of the lung (WHO 2007, pp. 12–13).

Asthma and COPD are very similar in presentation. Asthma is a disease of the airways due to chronic inflammation, hypersensitivity of the airways and a variable airway flow (Fréour 1987, NICE 2017). In both COPD and asthma, airflow may be obstructed due to over-secretion of mucus and airway thickening. In asthma there is broncho-constriction as the smooth muscle around the airways contracts, and there is bronchial inflammation that causes narrowing of the airways and oedema initiated by the immune response to allergens. The clinician should use history taking and spirometry testing to differentiate between the two conditions (NICE 2017).

COPD

COPD is an overarching term used to describe a chronic disorder, such as emphysema or bronchitis, where there is airflow obstruction (NICE 2011). There is an enhanced chronic inflammatory response in the airways to harmful inhalants such as cigarette smoke (GOLD 2015). It is thought to be one of the major causes of worldwide mortality (GOLD 2015).

Consider COPD as a differential diagnosis in anyone over 35 years old, who has a risk factor and presents with one or more of the following symptoms:

- Exertional breathlessness
- Chronic cough, regular sputum production
- Frequent winter 'bronchitis' wheeze.

These patients should be diagnosed as having COPD (BTS 2004, NICE 2017). This risk can also be due to passive smoking or pollution (BTS 2004, Yin *et al.* 2007).

Chronic obstructive pulmonary disease (COPD) is characterised as a chronic airflow limitation that is usually progressive and differs from asthma in that it is not fully reversible (GOLD 2015). However, there are some patients who have asthma-COPD overlap syndrome (ACOS) (Papaioannou *et al.* 2014). In this condition the smaller airways, which are <2 mm in internal diameter, are affected. At present there is no agreed definition for ACOS (GOLD 2015).

Inflammation is mainly due to the T cell co-receptor CD8 glycoprotein and macrophages in the bronchioles and alveoli (Kim & Rhee 2010, O'Shaughnessy *et al.* 1997). The damage within the airways is thought to affect the small airways and lung parenchyma (GOLD 2015). There is also tissue fibrosis and smooth muscle hypertrophy (airway remodelling) in the small airways which results in emphysema (GOLD 2015). Patients with COPD can present with bronchitic changes, emphysema or both.

The three main pathological changes that can occur in COPD are as follows:

- There is a loss of elasticity in the airways. The alveoli are damaged, resulting in loss of support and closure of small airways during expiration, as in emphysema (Duncan 2016, Postma & Rabe 2015).
- There is narrowing of the small airways due to inflammation, tissue damage and loss of elastic fibres (Black *et al.* 2008).
- The lumen of the small airways are obstructed with mucous secretions. There are large numbers of inflammatory infiltrates in the mucous secretory apparatus as in bronchitis (Postma & Rabe 2015). There is also mucus hypersecretion as there are goblet cells and enlarged submucosal glands due to chronic airway irritation (GOLD 2015). The pooling of the mucus can therefore lead to increased risk of infection.

Diagnosing COPD
A diagnosis of COPD should be considered in any patient over the age of 35 who has a history of:
- Exertional breathlessness
- Chronic cough
- Regular sputum production
- Frequent winter 'bronchitis'
- Wheeze.

(NICE 2010, Gold 2015)

However, there are also patients who are younger than 35 years who have the condition.

Other signs and symptoms of the disease are:
- Chronic breathlessness
- Fatigue
- Impaired immunity
- Low mood/Depression
- Polycythaemia
- Recurrent respiratory infections
- Weight loss and a low BMI, particularly in end-stage disease
- Exercise effort intolerance
- Waking at night
- Red flag symptoms:
  - Ankle swelling
  - Chest pain
  - Haemoptysis.

The GPN should seek advice from the practice mentor about the implications for patients who display any of these red flag symptoms.

Alpha-1 antitrypsin (A1AT) deficiency
Patients with COPD may also have the inherited condition alpha-1 antitrypsin (A1AT) deficiency, which means that they lack the A1AT glycoprotein. A1AT works in the lungs to mop up neutrophil elastase, thus preventing further cellular damage (Hill *et al.* 2000, Lomas 2006). It also digests damaged or aging lung cells and foreign particles (such as debris from smoking and bacteria). An A1AT deficiency prevents

the neutrophil elastase from being neutralised efficiently and therefore destroys the alveoli in the lungs (Lomas 2006). Once they lose their elasticity, the alveoli are left over-inflated and stretched and unable to expand and contract as normal. Holes then develop in their stretched walls, making them less able to fill with enough air and consequently even less effective, causing air trapping. A blood test is therefore offered to anyone with a history of alpha-1 antitrypsin deficiency or if it presents at a young age. The patient should be referred to a specialist centre to discuss the clinical management of this condition (NICE 2011).

Reader activity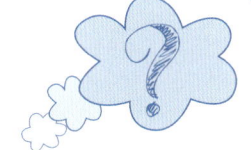

Mr Jackson is a 66-year-old retired builder who presents at the surgery during your flu clinic. He thinks he should have a flu vaccine, as he has the following symptoms:
- Chronic cough, regular sputum production
- Exertional breathlessness
- Frequent winter 'bronchitis' wheeze.

His past medical history is sparse.

Personal medical history: Appendix removed at 14 years old. He had a bout of pneumonia 4 years ago. Recurrent chest infections.

Social history: Married to Betty. They have 2 daughters and 3 grandchildren. His daughter has eczema. He lives in a two-storey house. He has a dog.

Medication: He has occasional hay fever. He takes one long-acting antihistamine daily. No OTC medication.

What tests do you need to arrange to help you determine his diagnosis?

Box 13.1: Reader activity – flu vaccine

Asthma

Asthma is a long-term respiratory condition that affects the airways in the lungs in children, young people and adults. The classic symptoms include breathlessness, tightness in the chest, coughing and wheezing (NICE 2017). In the UK, there are approximately 5.4 million people living with asthma, 1.1 million of whom are children (Asthma UK 2019). There are also around 1200 deaths a year from asthma, about 90 per cent of which are associated with preventable factors (Royal College of Physicians 2014).

Asthma is a disease of the airways and is caused by chronic inflammation and hypersensitivity of the airways (Kume *et al.* 2015, NICE 2012). There is an increase in CD4 lymphocyte-, eosinophil- and macrophages during the inflammatory response (Kim & Rhee 2010, Woodruff *et al.* 2009). There is also broncho-constriction as the smooth muscle around the airways contracts. This is due to bronchial narrowing, which can occur due to an increase in oedema triggered by the immune response to allergens (van den Berge 2011).

Diagnosing asthma

It is important to take a structured clinical history in patients you suspect may have asthma (NICE 2017). However, this will not enable you to make a diagnosis on its own. The physical examination should include examining patients to identify expiratory polyphonic wheeze and other signs of respiratory symptoms. However, these can be normal in patients with asthma and results should be interpreted within a holistic assessment (NICE 2018).

The following symptoms should also be considered:

- Wheeze, cough or breathlessness (including any daily/seasonal variation in these symptoms)
- Any triggers that make the symptoms worse
- The patient's personal or family history of any atopic disorders such as hay fever or eczema.

Spirometry

Spirometry is the recommended objective test, which can be carried out in practice, to help identify abnormalities in lung volumes and airflow (GOLD 2019, NICE 2018). Spirometry that is used for diagnosis should only be performed by people who have been trained and assessed to the Association for Respiratory Technology and Physiology (ARTP) or equivalent standards. Whatever their qualification, it needs to be from a recognised training body in the performance and interpretation of spirometry (ARTP 2013).

This is an important diagnostic test, as it can identify the presence of a post-bronchodilator FEV1/FVC <0.70 which confirms the presence of persistent airflow limitation or COPD (GOLD 2019, NICE 2018). The obstructive pattern has a reduction in maximum expiratory airflow relative to the maximum volume that can be expelled from the lung (a forced vital capacity). This indicates an obstructive problem due to the narrowed airways. In practice, the presence of airway obstruction is shown by a reduction in the FEV1/FVC ratio and a concave expiratory flow volume curve on the graph. So, in essence, the thickness of the small airways can be assessed by measuring the forced expiratory flow rates at 50 per cent of vital capacity (FEF 50 per cent) and at 25–75 per cent of vital capacity (FEF 25–75 per cent), and is a predictor of the severity of COPD (Bar-Yishay et al. 2003, GOLD 2015, Hogg et al. 2004). If a diagnosis of asthma is being considered, spirometry should be offered to adults, young people and children aged 5 and above.

Obstructive results show a reduction in maximum expiratory airflow relative to the maximum volume that can be expelled from the lung (the VC, measured as a forced manoeuvre) which reflects an obstructive ventilatory defect due to narrowed airways. In practice, the presence of airway obstruction is suggested by a reduced FEV1/FVC ratio, and the expiratory flow volume curve will appear concave. Several organisations have sought to simplify the diagnosis of airflow limitation by replacing the lower limit of normal (LLN) with a fixed cut-off of 0.70. However, since the FEV1/FVC ratio is dependent on age, height and sex, this leads to overdiagnosis of obstructive lung disease in elderly subjects, and to under-diagnosis in young subjects. Therefore, the presence of obstructive lung disease should be based on an FEV1/FVC ratio below the LLN.

Any condition that restricts airflow (such as interstitial lung disease) or extrinsic disorders (such as obesity, pregnancy, lung cancer or kyphoscoliosis) is characterised by a normal or increased FEV1/FVC ratio and a low FVC. The graph will have an expiratory flow volume curve that will appear convex. If this result is found on spirometry it will need to be reviewed by a senior clinician.

Bronchodilator reversibility (BDR)

This is part of the spirometry assessment and should be performed for adults with obstructive spirometry (FEV1/FVC ratio less than 70 per cent). An improvement in FEV1 of 12 per cent or more, with an increase in volume of 200ml or more, is considered a positive test (NICE 2017). This can also be performed in children and young people, aged 5 to 16. An improvement in FEV1 of 12 per cent or more is considered a positive test.

Peak expiratory flow variability
Peak flow variability should be assessed for 2 to 4 weeks in any adult if there is diagnostic uncertainty after initial assessment and a fractional exhaled nitric oxide (FeNO) test. This is regardless of whether they have had a normal spirometry or an obstructive spirometry, reversible airways obstruction (positive BDR) but a FeNO level of 39 ppb or less. A variation of 20 per cent is considered a positive test for asthma.

FeNO
Fractional exhaled nitric oxide (FeNO) should be obtained from a patient with suspected asthma if the equipment is available (NICE 2017). This is a non-invasive method of measuring airway inflammation and it can complement all other assessments (Dweik *et al.* 2011). Although NICE (2018) are clear about recommending FeNO testing, the BTS/SIGN (2016) lists FeNO as a potentially useful test but not essential. They specifically highlight its role in the investigation of people with an intermediate probability of asthma and without spirometric evidence of obstruction or reversibility (BTS/SIGN 2016, White *et al.* 2018).

Fractional exhaled nitric oxide
- A FeNO test should be offered to all adults (aged 17 and over) if a diagnosis of asthma is being considered. A positive test for the FeNO level is 40 parts per billion (ppb) or more.
- A FeNO test in children and young people (aged 5 to 16) can be obtained if there is diagnostic uncertainty after initial assessment and/or either: normal spirometry or obstructive spirometry with a negative bronchodilator reversibility (BDR) test. A FeNO level of 35 ppb or more is considered a positive test.

NB: A person's current smoking status can lower FeNO levels both acutely and cumulatively. However, a high level remains useful in supporting a diagnosis of asthma.

Box 13:2. Fractional exhaled nitric oxide

Other asthma tests
The following objective tests can also be done but they are usually performed after the formal diagnosis of asthma is made (NICE 2018):
- Skin prick tests to aeroallergens
- Serum total and specific ige
- Peripheral blood eosinophil count
- Exercise challenge (to adults aged 17 and over).

Subjective data

Subjective data can be obtained using a simple measure of breathlessness, such as the Modified British Medical Research Council (mMRC) Questionnaire, to measure breathlessness, although admittedly this only helps us measure one symptom of the disease (Bestall *et al.* 1999, Fletcher *et al.* 1959). There are also comprehensive disease-specific health-related quality of life or health status questionnaires such as the CRQ236 and SGRQ347. However, these can be too long to use in a consultation and the mMRC dyspnoea scale in Table 13.1 (below) may be more useful in practice.

Table 13.1: MRC dyspnoea scale

Grade	Degree of breathlessness related to activities
1	Not troubled by breathlessness except on strenuous exercise
2	Short of breath when hurrying or walking up a slight hill
3	Walks slower than contemporaries on level ground because of breathlessness, or has to stop for breath when walking at own pace
4	Stops for breath after walking about 100 metres or after a few minutes on level ground
5	Too breathless to leave the house, or breathless when dressing or undressing

(Adapted from Fletcher, C.M. et al. 1959)

Table 13.2 (below) lists the clinical features differentiating COPD and asthma (NICE 2018).

Table 13.2: Clinical features of asthma and COPD

Clinical feature	COPD	Asthma
Smoker or ex-smoker	Nearly all	Possibly
Symptoms under age 35	Rare	Often
Chronic productive cough	Common	Uncommon
Breathlessness	Persistent and progressive	Variable
Night-time waking with breathlessness and/or wheeze	Uncommon	Common
Significant diurnal or day-to-day variability of symptoms	Uncommon	Common

Managing respiratory disease

The aims of treatment for patients with respiratory disease are to reduce symptoms, prevent exacerbations and delay the progression of the disease using medication

(GOLD 2019). Management should also include lifestyle modifications such as smoking cessation as this reduces the progressive decline in lung function in COPD (NICE 2018). Other strategies should include vaccination against influenza and pneumococcal disease, increasing exercise tolerance, optimising mental wellbeing and education about self-management.

There are several effective medications available to prevent and control symptoms, improving patients' health status, and reducing the occurrence of COPD exacerbations by means of self-management (GOLD 2019, Pauwels *et al.* 2001). Personalised asthma action plans improve asthma control and COPD action plans reduce emergency health service use for patients with COPD. They are usually based on a traffic light system and give patients instructions on what to do in the event of worsening symptoms.

For asthma, the general principles of management are to increase or decrease treatment according to disease severity, enabling good control and minimising drug-related side-effects (Tidy 2016). The aim of treatment is to achieve control of asthma and its symptoms (NICE 2018), defined by the British National Formulary (NICE 2019a) as:

> *no daytime symptoms, no night-time awakening due to asthma, no asthma attacks, no need for rescue medication, no limitations on activity including exercise, normal lung function (in practical terms forced expiratory volume in 1 second (FEV1) and/or peak expiratory flow (PEF) > 80 per cent predicted or best), and minimal side-effects from treatment.*

There are a range of treatments for both conditions. For asthma these can be pharmacological such as bronchodilators, inhaled and oral steroids, antihistamines and anti-leukotrienes. Non- pharmacological approaches consist of trigger prevention, vaccines, breathing techniques, bronchothermaplasty and monoclonal antibodies. Medications commonly used for COPD are similar but first line treatment is bronchodilators (Suisse *et al.* 2018, GOLD 2018).

The inhaled medications most commonly used for respiratory conditions are:
- Short-acting beta agonists (SABAs)
- Short-acting muscarinic antagonists (SAMAs)
- Long-acting beta agonists (LABAs)
- Long-acting muscarinic antagonists (LAMAs)
- Inhaled steroids (IHSs).

The technique needed for each type of inhaler should be assessed on an annual basis. Some devices don't suit some patients. An example is the dry powder inhaler and the breath-actuated metered-dose inhaler, as they require an inspiratory flow of at least 20–30 L/min to activate the medication/ device (NHS Forth Valley 2013). The instructions come with each device and are available on both the MIM and BNF websites (see Box 13.5).

Bronchodilators

Beta2-receptor stimulating drugs (beta2-agonists) stimulate the beta2-receptors, causing the airway smooth muscles to relax, creating bronchodilation (Duncan 2017). They are effective, giving relief for both asthma and COPD patients. Selective beta2 agonists can come in the form of a standard inhaler pMDI (pressurised metered-dose inhaler). An alternative choice of inhaler device should be based on patient preference and assessment of use such as Terbutaline (inhaled and nebulised) (NICE 2019a).

Longer-acting beta2 agonists include Salmeterol and Formoterol. Indacaterol and Olodaterol (Striverdi Respimat®) are licensed for maintenance of COPD (NICE 2019a). It is worth noting that longer-acting beta2 agonists should not be used for the relief of an acute asthma attack. They are only indicated in chronic asthma (NICE 2017). However, symptoms of COPD may be alleviated by an inhaled short-acting beta2 agonist or a short-acting antimuscarinic bronchodilator as a first-line treatment (BTS/SIGN 2016).

Antimuscarinic bronchodilators

The short acting antimuscarinic is Ipratropium but it should be stopped if the patient is started on the longer-acting Tiotropium. Tiotropium can be prescribed in two different devices. The strength and the dose are different for the Tiotropium Respimat® device compared to the Handihaler® as the Respimat® inhaler strength is 2.5 micrograms Tiotropium per puff. The recommended dose for adults is 5 micrograms Tiotropium, given as two puffs from the Respimat® inhaler once daily, at the same time of the day.

In patients with asthma, the following can be prescribed:

- Aclidinium Eklira®
- Glycopyrronium Seebri®
- Umeclidinium Incruse Ellipta®.

Inhaled steroids (IHSs)

Inhaled steroids are considered as routine maintenance medications or preventive therapy. A low dose of inhaled corticosteroid should therefore be started in patients who present with any one of the following:

- Using an inhaled short-acting beta2 agonist 3 times a week or more
- Symptomatic 3 times a week or more
- Waking at night due to asthma symptoms at least once a week.

BTS/SIGN (2016) also recommend initiation of HIS treatment for patients who have had an asthma attack in the last 2 years. However, inhaled steroids are not considered as a first-line treatment for COPD. A trial of a high-dose inhaled corticosteroid or an oral corticosteroid is recommended only for patients with moderate or severe COPD or those patients who have had two or more exacerbations in the past year (BTS/SIGN 2016, NICE 2018). Other anti-inflammatories include antagonists such as montelukast, non-steroidal anti-inflammatories like sodium cromoglicate and PDE4 inhibitors like roflumilast (MIMS 2018).

Each area will have a prescribing formulary. The types of corticosteroid most commonly prescribed in practice are as follows:

- Beclomethasone – Budelin
- Beclomethasone dipropionate – Clenil* + Qvar. Easy haler/pMDI
- Budesonide – Pulmicort. Turbohaler/Easy haler
- Ciclesonide – Alvesco
- Clenil
- Fluticasone – Flixotide. pMDI/Evohaler/Accuhaler
- Mometasone – Asmanex (Twist haler)
- Budesonide with formeterol – Fobumix
- Easy haler/Turbohaler/Duoresp spiromax
- Budesonide with formeterol – Fostair – MDI/Next haler.

Combination preparations

There are several combination products, which include LAMA/LABA, LABA/ICS and SABA/SAMA formulations (MIMS 2018). The prescribing of (leukotriene receptor) LTRA after ICS is potentially the most contentious and problematic issue in the various guidelines. The BTS/SIGN (2016) guidelines suggest that low-dose ICS should be stepped up to the next treatment level with the addition of long-acting beta-agonists (LABAs). This is in line with international guidelines, such as GOLD (2019). However, NICE (2018) favour LTRA, even though LABA is known to be the more effective treatment for asthma (White *et al*. 2018).

For patients with COPD, long-acting beta2 agonists (LABAs), in combination with ICS and long-acting muscarinic antagonists (LAMAs), are the recommended initial maintenance treatment (Suissa *et al*. 2018). However, based on their longitudinal study which ran from 2002 to 2015, Suissa *et al*. (2018) suggest that there was an increased risk of pneumonia associated with the ICS component of the combination and that initiation with a LAMA should be preferred in patients with blood eosinophil concentrations of less than 4 per cent.

Maintenance and reliever therapy (MART)
MART regimes are combination inhalers with a combination of IHS and bronchodilator and they have been shown to reduce exacerbations in adults (BTS/SIGN 2016, NICE 2017). In fact, NICE recommends a MART regimen for people with asthma 'uncontrolled on a low dose of ICS/LABA, with or without an LTRA' if the maintenance ICS dose should continue to be 'low' (NICE 2017). Examples include the drugs Fostair (Formeterol/Beclomethasone) and Symbicort (Budesonide/Formeterol).

Leukotriene-receptor antagonists
The leukotrienes used to treat asthma are from the second group of cysteinyl-leukotrienes which act on eosinophil and mast cell-induced bronchoconstriction. They bind to the selective receptors on the bronchial smooth muscle in the airways, preventing leukotriene release from mast cells and eosinophils. This in turn prevents bronchoconstriction, mucus secretion and oedema. One example of a leukotriene-based drug is Singulair (Montelukast) which is prescribed for the treatment of asthma in adults and children ≥12 months (NICE 2019a).

Xanthines
Xanthines are classified as oral bronchodilators as they are thought to relax the smooth muscle and increase diaphragm contractility when used for patients with asthma and COPD (NICE 2018). Aminophylline (Phyllocontin®) m/r and Theophylline (patient's usual brand) m/r are commonly used in the UK (NICE 2018, NICE 2019a). Theophylline is used at step 3 of the nationally agreed treatment algorithm or as an add-in asthma management (NICE 2018). It should be considered only for patients in whom other treatments have failed to control symptoms adequately.

These drugs have some unpleasant side effects so not everyone wants to continue taking them for long periods. These side effects include nausea and vomiting, insomnia, cardiac arrhythmias, seizures and hypokalaemia (BNF 2018). The liver enzymes responsible for theophylline metabolism are also inhibited by a range of drugs, including macrolides such as erythromycin, quinolones and ciprofloxacin. In these situations, the patient must be monitored closely.

It may be helpful to measure plasma theophylline concentration, and this is essential if aminophylline is to be given to patients who are already taking theophylline because serious side effects (such as convulsions and arrhythmias) can occasionally precede other symptoms of toxicity. If continuing previous theophylline therapy, continue with the brand of theophylline the patient is stabilised on. Tobacco smoking increases the metabolism of theophylline. Smoking cessation can cause theophylline plasma levels to rise.

Phosphodiesterase type-4 inhibitors

Roflumilast (Daxas) is recommended as an add-on to bronchodilator therapy for treating severe chronic obstructive pulmonary disease in adults with chronic bronchitis, providing certain criteria are met. The *MHRA Drug Safety Update January 2013* detailed that there was a risk of suicidal behaviour associated with the use of roflumilast and so it should be avoided in patients with previous or existing psychiatric symptoms and treatment should be discontinued if new or worsening symptoms are identified (MHRA 2014, NICE 2019b).

Mucolytics

Mucolytic drug therapy should be considered in COPD patients with a chronic cough productive of sputum (GOLD 2018). It can be continued if there is symptomatic improvement after 4 to 6 weeks and only continued in patients where there is clear symptomatic improvement (NICE 2019a). Mucolytics should also be used with caution in those with a history of peptic ulceration because they may disrupt the gastric mucosal barrier (NICE 2019a). Often the first drug of choice is Carbocisteine capsules 375mg or oral solution 250mg/5ml (NICE 2019a).

Inhaler devices

Short-acting reliever inhalers:

- Metered dose inhalers (MDIs) – Ventolin, Airomir and Salamol
- Breath actuated inhalers (BAIs) – Easi-breathe, Airmax and Autohaler
- Dry powder inhalers (DPIs) – Accuhaler (usually blue in colour).

Long-acting reliever inhalers:

- Long-acting beta agonists (LABAs) – Serevent Evohaler (Salmeterol), Vertine Metered-dose inhalers (Salmeterol), Formoterol Easyhaler (Formoterol), Oxis Turbohaler (Formoterol) and Foradil Dry Powder Inhaler (Formoterol)

These are generally green in colour.

Long acting anti-muscarinics (LAMAs):

- Seebri: glycopyrronium bromide, 55mcg, once daily
- Incruse Elipta: umeclidium bromide, 65mg, once daily
- Spiriva respimat: tiotropium, 2.5mg, once daily, pressurised device
- Handihaler: tiotropium bromide, 18mcg, once daily
- Braltus: tiotropium bromide 10mcg.

Preventer inhalers:
- Metered-dose inhalers (MDIs) – Beclomethasone, Qvar, Clenil
- Breath-actuated inhalers (BAIs) – Easibreath, Airmax, Autohaler
- Dry powder inhalers (DPIs) – Accuhaler (usually brown in colour)
- These inhaled corticosteroids are similar in efficacy and adverse effect profile. NB: Qvar® and Clenil Modulite® (beclometasone CFC-free brands) should be prescribed by brand name as they are not equivalent in dose and are not interchangeable. The drug Qvar® has extra-fine particles and is therefore twice as potent as the Clenil Modulite® (NICE 2019a).

Combination inhalers:
- Salmeterol + Fluticasone = Aerivio Spiromax
- Seretide – Accuhaler + Easyhaler/Sirdupla/Sereflo-pMDI
- Fucacombe – Easyhaler. Combisal – pMDI. Aloflute – pDMI
- Airflusal – MDI
- Formeterol + Aclidinium = Duaklir (Genuair)
- Formeterol + Beclomethasone: Fostair. pMDI. NEXThaler
- Formeterol + Budesonide = DuoResp (Spiromax). Symbicort – turbohaler, Fobumix – Easyhaler
- Formeterol fumarate + fluticasone propionate. Flutiform: pMDI. Flutiform K haler
- Indacterol+ Glycopyrronium = Ultibro (breezhaler).
- Olodaterol + tiotropium = Spiriva (Handihaler. Respimat)
- Spiolto (Respimat)
- Vilanterol + Fluticasone = Relvar (Ellipta)
- Vilanterol + umeclidinium = Anoro (Ellipta)
- Salbutamol + Ipratropium = Aerivio/Sereflo: (Spiromax).

Box 13.3: Inhaler devices

Summary

In summary, we have seen that, although COPD and asthma are obstructive diseases, their management can vary. It is therefore important to gain the correct information at diagnosis. This chapter has provided an introduction to the topic and you will need to familiarise yourself with national and local guidelines. It will also take time to remember all the inhaler devices and the medications used in each of them.

> ### Reader activity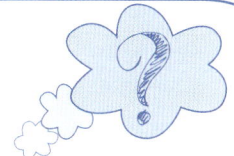
>
> What tests and assessments do you need to arrange in order to determine Mr Jackson's diagnosis and the best management of his condition?
> **Further tests should include:**
> - Chest radiograph to exclude other pathologies
> - Full blood count (FBC) to identify anaemia or polycythaemia
> - Body mass index (BMI) calculated – may need dietician assessment
> - Mood assessment
> - Medication review
> - Inhaler assessment if prescribed inhaler devices
> - Assessment of smoking, with smoking cessation advice if necessary
> - Immunisation history including influenza and pneumovax history
> - ECG
> - To assess cardiac status if features of cor pulmonale (oedema) are present
> - Pulse oximetry
> - Sputum culture – to identify organisms if sputum is persistently present and purulent.

Box 13.4: Answers to reader activity – flu vaccine

Resources

Asthma UK: https://www.asthma.org.uk

MIMS inhaler device guide: https://www.mims.co.uk/table-asthma-copd-preparations-compatible-devices/respiratory-system/article/1427948

The Association for Respiratory Technology and Physiology: www.artp.org.uk/

The Electronic Medicines Compendium: https://www.medicines.org.uk/emc

Box 13.5: Resources

References

Association for Respiratory Technology & Physiology (ARTP) (2013). *A Guide to Performing Quality Assured Diagnostic Spirometry.* http://www.artp.org.uk/en/professional/artp-standards/index.cfm/QADS%20Apr%202013 (last accessed 28.1.2019).

Asthma UK (2019). https://www.asthma.org.uk/ (last accessed 20.2.2019).

Bar-Yishay, E., Amiray, I. & Goldberg, S. (2003). Comparison of Maximal Mid Expiratory Flow Rate and Forced Expiratory Flow at 50 per cent of Vital Capacity in children. *Chest Journal.* 123.3.731

Bestall, J., Paula, E., Garroda, R., Garnhama, R., Jones, P. & Wedzichaa, J. (1999). Usefulness of the Medical Research Council (MRC) dyspnoea scale as a measure of disability in patients with chronic obstructive pulmonary disease. *Thorax.* **54**, 581–86.

Black, P., Ching, P., Beaumont, S., Ranasinghe, G., Taylor, G. & Merrilees, M. (2008). Changes in elastic fibres in the small airways and alveoli in COPD. *European Respiratory Journal.* **31**, 998–1004; DOI: 10.1183/09031936.00017207

British Thoracic Society (BTS) (2004). *Update of BTS pneumonia guidelines: what's new?* http://dx.doi.org/10.1136/thx.2004.024992 (last accessed 28.1.2019).

BTS/SIGN (2016). *Health Improvement Scotland. BTS/SIGN. British guideline on the management of asthma. SIGN 153.* https://www.sign.ac.uk/sign-153-british-guideline-on-the-management-of-asthma.html (last accessed 28.1.2019).

Duncan, D. (2016). Chronic obstructive pulmonary disease: an overview. *British Journal of Nursing.* **25**(7), 360–66.

Dweik, R., Boggs, P., Erzurum, S., Irvin, C., Leigh, M., Lundberg, O., Olin, A., Plummer, A., Taylor, D. and on behalf of the American Thoracic Society Committee on Interpretation of Exhaled Nitric Oxide Levels (FeNO) for Clinical Applications (2011). An Official ATS Clinical Practice Guideline: Interpretation of Exhaled Nitric Oxide Levels (FeNO) for Clinical Applications. *American Journal of Respiratory and Critical Care Medicine.* **184**, 5.

Fletcher, C.M., Elmes, P.C., Fairbairn, M.B. *et al.* (1959) The significance of respiratory symptoms and the diagnosis of chronic bronchitis in a working population. *British Medical Journal.* **2**, 257–66.

Fréour, P. (1987). Definition of asthma. *Chest Journal.* **91**(6), Supplement191S.

Global Initiative for Chronic Obstructive Lung Disease (GOLD) (2008). *Striving to improve diagnosis, prevention and management of COPD across the globe.* http://www.goldcopd.com (last accessed 28.1.2019).

Global Initiative for Chronic Obstructive Lung Disease (GOLD) (2019). *Global strategy for the diagnosis, management, and prevent of chronic obstructive pulmonary disease.* https://goldcopd.org/wp-content/uploads/2018/11/GOLD-2019-v1.7-FINAL-14Nov2018-WMS.pdf (last accessed 27.2.2019).

Hill, K., Goldstein, R., Guyatt, G., Blouin, M., Tan, W., Davis, L., Heels-Ansdell, D., Erak, M., Bragaglia, P., Tamari, I., Hodder, R. & Stanbrook, M. (2010). Prevalence and underdiagnosis of chronic obstructive pulmonary disease among patients at risk in primary care. *Canadian Medical Association Journal.* **182**(7) 673–78; DOI: https://doi.org/10.1503/cmaj.091784 (last accessed 28.1.2019).

Hogg, J.C., Chu, F., Utokaparch, S., Woods, R., Elliott, W..M, Buzatu, L., *et al.* (2004). The nature of small-airway obstruction in chronic obstructive pulmonary disease. *New England Journal of Medicine.* **350**, 2645–53.

Kim, R. & Rhee, Y. (2010). Overlap between asthma and COPD: Where the two diseases converge. The Korean Academy of Asthma, Allergy and Clinical Immunology. *Allergy Asthma and Immunology Research.* **2**(4), 209–14. English. https://doi.org/10.4168/aair.2010.2.4.209 (last accessed 28.1.2019).

Kume, H., Fukunaga, K. & Oguma, T. (2015). Research and development of bronchodilators for asthma and COPD with a focus on G protein/KCa channel linkage and β2-adrenergic intrinsic efficacy. *Pharmacology and Therapeutics.* **156**, 75–89.

Lomas, D. A. (2006). The selective advantage of α1-antitrypsin deficiency. *American Journal of Respiratory and Critical Care Medicine,* **173**(10), 1072–77.

MHRA (2014). Roflumilast (Daxas): risk of suicidal behaviour. https://www.gov.uk/government/organisations/medicines-and-healthcare-products-regulatory-agency (last accessed 27.02.2019)

MIMS (2018). *Asthma and COPD preparations and compatible devices.* https://www.mims.co.uk/asthma-copd-preparations-compatible-devices/respiratory-system/article/882435 (last accessed 28.1.2019).

NICE (2010). *Chronic obstructive pulmonary disease in over 16s: diagnosis and management. Clinical guideline [CG101].* https://www.nice.org.uk/guidance/CG101/chapter/1-Guidance#diagnosing-copd (last accessed 28.1.2019).

NICE (2018). *Asthma: diagnosis, monitoring and chronic asthma management. NICE guideline [NG80].* https://www.nice.org.uk/guidance/qs25 (last accessed 28.1.2019).

NICE (2019a). *Asthma, chronic description of condition.* https://bnf.nice.org.uk/treatment-summary/asthma-chronic.html (last accessed 20/02/2019).

NICE (2019b). ROFLUMILAST. https://bnf.nice.org.uk/drug/roflumilast.html (last accessed 20.02.2019).

NHS Forth Valley (2013). *Inhaler assessment information. Guidelines for the management of asthma. 8.1. NHS Forth Valley.* https://docplayer.net/21035797-Nhs-forth-valley-guideline-for-the-management-of-asthma.html (last accessed 28.1.2019).

O'Shaughnessy, T., Ansari, T., Barnes, N. & Jeffery, P. (1997). Inflammation in bronchial biopsies of subjects with chronic bronchitis: inverse relationship of CD8+ T lymphocytes with FEV1. *American Journal of Respiratory and Critical Care Medicine.* **155**, 3. https://doi.org/10.1164/ajrccm.155.3.9117016 (last accessed 28.1.2019).

Papaioannou, M., Pitsiou, G., Manika, K., Kontou., P., Zarogoulidis, P., Sichletidis, L. *et al.* (2014). COPD Assessment Test: A simple tool to evaluate disease severity and response to treatment. *Journal of Chronic Obstructive Pulmonary Disease.* **11**(5), 489–95

Pauwels, R.A., Buist, A.S., Calverley, P.M., *et al.* (2001). Global strategy for the diagnosis, management, and prevention of chronic obstructive pulmonary disease. NHLBI/WHO Global Initiative for Chronic Obstructive Lung Disease (GOLD) Workshop summary. *American Journal of Respiratory Critical Care Medicine.* **163**, 1256–76.

Postma, D. & Rabe, K. (2015). The asthma-COPD overlap syndrome. *New England Journal of Medicine.* **373**(13),1241–49. doi: 10.1056/NEJMra1411863.

Royal College of Physicians (2014). *National Review of Asthma Deaths.* https://www.rcplondon.ac.uk/projects/national-review-asthma-deaths (last accessed 28.1.2019).

Suissa, S., Dell'Aniello, S. & Ernst, P. (2018). Comparative effectiveness of LABA-ICS versus LAMA as initial treatment in COPD targeted by blood eosinophils: a population-based cohort study. *The Lancet.* **6** (11), 855–62.

Tidy, C. (2016). *Management of Adult Asthma.* https://patient.info/doctor/Management-Of-Adult-Asthma (last accessed 28.1.2019).

White, J., Paton, J., Niven, R. & Pinnock, H., on behalf of the British Thoracic Society (BTS) (2018). *Guidelines for the diagnosis and management of asthma: a look at the key differences between BTS/SIGN and NICE.* https://www.brit-thoracic.org.uk/media/382969/thoraxjnl-2017-211189.pdf (last accessed 28.1.2019).

Woodruff, P., Modrek, B., Choy, D., Jia, G., Abbas, A., Ellwanger, A., Arron, J., Koth, L. & Fahy, J. (2009). T-helper Type 2–driven inflammation defines major subphenotypes of asthma. *American Journal of Respiratory Critical Care Medicine.* **180**(5), 388–95. https://www.ncbi.nlm.nih.gov/pmc/articles/PMC2742757/ (last accessed 28.1.2019).

World Health Organization (WHO) (2007). *Living a normal life with asthma.* http://www.who.int/features/2007/asthma/en/ (last accessed 28.1.2019).

Yin, P., Jiang, C., Cheng, K., Lam, T., Lam, K., *et al.* (2007). Passive smoking exposure and risk of COPD among adults in China: the Guangzhou Biobank Cohort Study. *The Lancet.* **370**(9589), 751–57.

Chapter 14

Chronic kidney disease

Evelyn Walton

Introduction

Chronic kidney disease (CKD) is an abnormality of kidney function or structure that is present for more than 3 months, with implications for health (NICE 2014). It is a gradual impairment in kidney function, which over time can progress to end-stage renal disease. With careful management and treatment of underlying causes, this process can be slowed or even reversed (GAIN 2015). The management of CKD is central to the role of the GPN, and an understanding of this condition will directly affect the quality of care provided.

Prevalence

The prevalence of CKD is estimated to be 8.5 per cent in adults (NICE 2014). This increases with age, with 20 per cent of men and 25 per cent of women between the age of 65 and 75 years estimated to have some degree of it (Mendes 2015). As our population ages, the prevalence will continue to rise.

Causes

Specific causes include conditions such as diabetes, atheromatous renal vascular disease, glomerulonephritis, pyelonephritis and polycystic kidney disease. For many patients, no specific cause is identified, and the CKD is presumed to be related to hypertensive or ischaemic kidney damage, both of which are more common with advancing age (GAIN 2015).

Signs and symptoms

CKD is usually discovered by chance, following a routine blood or urine test. Specific symptoms usually only develop in severe CKD. These include anorexia, nausea, vomiting, fatigue, pruritus, peripheral oedema, dyspnoea, insomnia, muscle cramps, pulmonary oedema, polyuria and headache (Lowth 2013).

Prognosis

CKD can progress to end-stage renal disease in a small proportion of people – about 2 per cent (NICE 2014). In fact, people with CKD are roughly 20 times more likely to die of cardiovascular disease than to progress to end-stage renal disease. The all-cause mortality rate for CKD is up to 60 per cent higher than that of the general population (NICE 2016).

However, there is evidence that treatment can slow both the progression of CKD and the associated cardiovascular risk (Jameson *et al.* 2014). Early diagnosis and intervention produce the most dramatic benefits (Lowth 2013). All patients at risk of CKD should be offered screening for this reason – the earlier the intervention, the greater the impact.

Screening for CKD

Patients at risk of CKD should be offered assessment of their estimated glomerular filtration rate (eGFR) and urine albumin:creatinine ratio (ACR) (GAIN 2015). Offer testing for patients with the following risk factors:

- Acute kidney injury
- Cardiovascular disease
- Diabetes
- Structural renal tract disease, recurrent renal calculi or prostatic hypertrophy
- Multisystem diseases, e.g. systemic lupus erythematosus (SLE), rheumatoid arthritis or sarcoidosis
- Family history of end-stage kidney disease
- Haematuria
- Those taking nephrotoxic drugs such as angiotensin-converting enzyme (ACE) inhibitors, angiotensin11 receptor antagonists (ARBs), ciclosporin, diuretics, lithium and long-term nonsteroidal anti-inflammatory drugs (NSAIDs)
- Obesity with metabolic syndrome (NICE 2016).

Advise the patient not to eat meat for at least 12 hours before measuring eGFR and interpret with caution if the person has a large muscle mass, or if they are pregnant, oedematous or malnourished. The urine ACR should be an early morning urine sample (NICE 2016).

Diagnosis and classification of CKD

CKD is diagnosed when tests have persistently (>3 months) shown the presence of proteinuria or a reduction in kidney function. Diagnose if the eGFR is persistently less than 60, and/or the urinary ACR is persistently greater than 3mg/mmol (NICE 2016). NICE has adopted the US National Kidney Foundation Kidney Disease Outcomes Quality Initiative (NKF-KDOQI) classification, which describes five stages of CKD (Inker *et al.* 2014). Table 14.1 (below) recognises that an increased ACR and a decreased eGFR are each associated with a higher risk of adverse outcomes, and that if both are present the risk is multiplied (Inker *et al.* 2014).

Table 14.1: Prognosis of CKD by GFR and albuminuria categories

				Albuminaria categories Description and range		
				A1	A2	A3
				Normal to mildly increased	Moderately increased	Severely increased
				<30mg/g <3mg/mmol	30–299mg/g 3–29mg/mmol	≥300mg/g ≥30mg/mmol
GFR categories (ml/min/1.73m²) Description and range	G1	Normal or high	≥90	Green	Yellow	Orange
	G2	Mildly decreased	60–90	Green	Yellow	Orange
	G3a	Mildly to moderately decreased	45–59	Yellow	Orange	Red
	G3b	Moderately to severely decreased	30–44	Orange	Red	Red
	G4	Severely decreased	15–29	Red	Red	Red
	G5	Kidney failure	<15	Red	Red	Red

Green: low risk (if no other markeers of kidney disease, no CKD); Yellow: moderately increased risk; Orange: high risk; Red: very high risk.
KDIGO 2012

Managing CKD

The aims of CKD management are to prevent disease progression and its associated risks.

Patients should have an annual cardiovascular risk assessment using a recognised tool such as the JBS3 risk calculator (JBS 2014). Lipid profile is assessed, as well as BMI, exercise, alcohol and smoking. There should also be a review of interventions to reduce cardiovascular risk (NICE 2014):

- Statins lower death and major cardiovascular events by 20 per cent in people with CKD (Palmer *et al.* 2014). Offer Atorvastatin 20mg initially.
- Antiplatelet drugs are beneficial for secondary prevention of cardiovascular disease, but there is an increased risk of bleeding (NICE 2014).
- Blood pressure should be kept below – 140/80mmHg, or 130/80mmhg if the patient has diabetes (NICE 2014).

An ACE inhibitor or ARB should be used if there is diabetes and the ACR is 3mg/mmol or more, or if there is hypertension and an ACR of 30mg/mmol or more, or if the ACR is greater than 70mg/mmol. ACE inhibitors and ARBs should not be used in combination (NICE 2016). Serum potassium levels should be checked prior to starting these drugs, and between 1 and 2 weeks after starting or increasing the dose (Lowth 2013).

All patients with stage 4–5 CKD should have their body weight and BMI recorded regularly and receive dietary advice to restrict their sodium intake to <2.4g/daily. Some dietary restriction of sodium and potassium is appropriate, if patients can tolerate this. The risk of hyperkalaemia may be reduced by avoiding some fruits, coffee and chocolate (Ramlan 2015). A low-protein diet is not recommended (NICE 2016).

Stopping smoking reduces the risk of CKD, and continuation of smoking has been shown to increase the risk of disease progression (NICE 2016). Smoking cessation is therefore a priority in managing these high-risk patients. Alcohol intake is linked to hypertension and cardiovascular disease so patients should be encouraged to drink sensibly (SIGN 2017).

Patients with CKD may be very anxious about their diagnosis, assuming that they will end up on renal dialysis. It is important to explain that mild CKD is common and is unlikely to progress. The link between CKD and cardiovascular disease needs to be explained in a way that the patient can understand. The patient must make informed choices about their lifestyle and treatments aimed at reducing this risk. The JBS3 calculator provides a visual guide to demonstrate how modifying their risk factors (e.g. stopping smoking) can reduce their personal risk (JBS 2014). Lifestyle changes must be realistic and patient-led, with the GPN negotiating through motivational interviewing (William & Rollnick 2013).

Renal function must be monitored in patients with CKD, and the frequency of monitoring should be tailored to the individual patient. An accelerated progression of CKD is indicated by a sustained decrease in estimated eGFR of 25 per cent or more within a year, or a sustained decrease in eGFR of 15ml/min per year (NICE 2016).

Bloods should be monitored – this includes a full blood picture to identify renal anaemia and serum calcium, phosphate, vitamin D and parathyroid hormone to check for bone disease (NICE 2016).

Referral to a nephrology specialist is normally required if:

- The eGFR is less than 30
- There is a sustained decrease of eGFR of 25 per cent or more within a year and a change in eGFR category
- The ACR is above 70mg/mmol (unless it is caused by diabetes and is being treated)
- The ACR is over 30mg/mmol, together with persistent haematuria, after infection has been ruled out.

Summary

CKD is a common presentation in General Practice and it is likely to become more prevalent as more patients are living with it than dying with it. Support and compassion are paramount when caring for these high- risk patients.

The challenges for the GPN are early identification of patients with CKD and ensuring a good quality of life for these patients, with an appropriate management plan. This patient group needs appropriate lifestyle advice and pharmacological therapies, which require continued effort and engagement from the GPN to help them make lasting changes.

Resources

NHS Choices: https://www.nhs.uk/conditions/kidney-disease/

Kidney Research UK: https://www.kidneyresearchuk.org/health-information/chronic-kidney-disease

Box 14.1: Resources

References

GAIN (2015). Guidelines and Audit Implementation Network. *Northern Ireland Guidelines for Management of Chronic Kidney Disease.* https://rqia.org.uk/RQIA/files/6d/6d79bfd8-8d75-42a5-a24d-6487e443c001.pdf (last accessed 29.1.2019).

Inker, L., Astor, B., Fox, C. & Isakova, T. (2014). KDOQI US Commentary on the 2012 KDIGO Clinical Practice Guideline for the Evaluation and Management of CKD. *American Journal of Kidney Disease.* **63**(5), 713–35.

Jameson, K., Jick, S. & Hagberg, K.W. (2014). Prevalence and management of chronic kidney disease in primary care patients in the UK. *International Journal of Clinical Practice.* **68**(9), 1110–21.

JBS (2014). Joint British Societies for the prevention of cardiovascular disease (JBS3). http://www.jbs3risk.com/pages/Who_calculator_For.htm (last accessed 29.1.2019).

Lowth, M. (2013). Chronic Kidney Disease. *Practice Nurse.* **43**(1), 34–39.

Mendes, A. (2015). Chronic Kidney Disease: supporting at-risk and diagnosed patients. *British Journal of Community Nursing.* **20**(2), 97–99.

NICE (2014). *Chronic Kidney Disease in Adults: assessment and management.* https://www.nice.org.uk/guidance/cg182 (last accessed 29.1.2019).

NICE (2016) *Chronic Kidney Disease – not diabetic. Clinical Knowledge Summary Revised May 2016* https://cks.nice.org.uk/chronic-kidney-disease-not-diabetic (last accessed 29.1.2019).

Palmer, S.C., Navaneethan, S.D. & Craig, J.C. (2014). HMG CoA reductase inhibitors (statins) for people with chronic kidney disease nit requiring dialysis. *Cochrane Database Systematic Review.* 5, CD007784. doi: 10.1002/14651858. CD007784.pub2.

Ramlan, G. (2015) Dietary challenges in patients with diabetes and chronic kidney disease. *Journal of Renal Nursing.* **7**(2), 58–63.

(SIGN) (2017) SIGN 149. *Risk estimation and the prevention of cardiovascular disease.* http://www.sign.ac.uk/assets/sign149.pdf (last accessed 29.1.2019).

William, R. & Rollnick, S. (2013) *Motivational Interviewing, Helping People Change (Applications of Motivational Interviewing).* 3rd edn. New York: Guildford Press.

Chapter 15

Coronary heart disease

Evelyn Walton

Introduction

Coronary heart disease (CHD) is the most common type of cardiovascular disease (CVD). It occurs when coronary arteries become narrowed due to a build-up of atheroma, a fatty material within the walls. It is the leading cause of death worldwide, with 2.3 million people living with CHD in the UK (Quality Outcome Framework 2017).

In the UK, nearly 1 in 7 women and 1 in 12 men die from CHD, averaging 1 death every 8 minutes (BHF 2018a). Most of these deaths are caused by myocardial infarction, with 1 patient presenting to hospital every 3 minutes (BHF 2018a).

The GPN has a significant role to play in both the prevention and management of CHD. Primary health care professionals are in an ideal position to use their knowledge and skills to improve the health and wellbeing of the patient in general practice. There is an expectation that every nurse should be a health-promoting practitioner (Public Health England 2018, Nursing and Midwifery Council 2015).

Working out cardiovascular risk

The National Institute for Clinical Excellence (2014a) recommends that patients should be treated if they have a 10 per cent (or higher) risk of developing CVD. This includes lipid modification (NICE 2014a).

The JBS3 Risk Calculator has been designed primarily for use by doctors and other healthcare practitioners, such as nurses (JBS 2014a). It is intended as a tool to communicate a patient's risk of cardiovascular disease and show the benefits that interventions can have in reducing their risk of CVD. There are several screens within the risk calculator, giving clinicians a choice of how to communicate risk of CVD to their patient.

The JBS3 Risk Calculator should *not* be used for patients known to have existing CVD, where treatment and health care professional advice should be followed according to established recommendations.

The JBS3 Risk Calculator must be used *with caution* for patients with certain high-risk conditions, such as high blood pressure, diabetes and chronic kidney disease, as specific drug treatments and other recommendations may already be indicated in these conditions (JBS 2014b). However, the Risk Calculator may be of additional help in highlighting the high risk and the benefits of an intervention. Note also that when total cholesterol exceeds 7.5mmol/L the calculator will highlight the possibility of familial hypercholesterolaemia, for which further assessment is indicated (JBS 2014a).

Patients must understand their personal cardiovascular risk in order to make informed choices about their treatment and any lifestyle interventions needed to reduce their risk. The JBS3 calculator gives them 'actual heart age' and demonstrates how modifying their risk factors can improve their health status.

The GPN must have an awareness of contributory risk factors for CHD. These can be broken into unmodifiable and modifiable risk factors.

Unmodifiable risk factors:
- Age (>45yrs men, >55yrs women)
- Gender (Male)
- Family history of early heart disease
- Race (African or Asian ancestry).

These are the risk factors that we are unable to change or reduce, but it is important for the GPN to be aware of them in order to identify those patients who are at higher risk from CHD.

Modifiable risk factors:
- Overweight/obesity
- Sedentary lifestyle
- Hypertension
- Hypercholesterolaemia
- Smoking
- Alcohol and drug misuse
- Diabetes.

Premature death rates from CHD have fallen consistently since 2000 due not only to medical treatments, but also smoking cessation, increased activity and reducing cholesterol levels (Loades 2017).

Behaviour change is a complex process and advice to the patient needs to be specific, achievable, and based on what they feel is their priority. The change needs to be realistic and patient-led. If we tell a patient what to do, they will most likely not do it (Miller & Rollnick 2013). This is an essential part of human behaviour, yet we as health care professionals frequently fall into this trap of 'telling' rather than negotiating through motivational interviewing (William & Rollnick 2013).

Overweight/obesity

More than 40 per cent of males and 30 per cent of females are classified as obese, with 26 per cent of men and 27 per cent of women overweight in England (NHS Digital 2018). It is predicted that 60 per cent of men and 50 per cent of women will be obese by 2050. Obesity is more dangerous than smoking, reducing life expectancy by up to 13 years (Butland *et al.* 2007).

Long-term studies indicate that obesity not only relates to but independently predicts coronary atherosclerosis (Garrison & Castelli 1985). This relationship appears to exist for men and women with minimal increases in body mass index, with up to a 72 per cent increased risk of CHD for individuals with a BMI between 25 and 29 (Rabkin & Matthewson 1977).

A diet that is low in saturated fat helps to reduce CHD risk. Oily fish may have a role in reducing risk but Omega-3 fatty acid supplements should not be offered. Increased fruit and vegetable consumption is recommended for the entire population to reduce risk (SIGN 2017). NICE have issued dietary advice which includes choosing wholegrain varieties of starchy foods, reducing sugar intake and eating at least five portions of fruit and vegetables per day. Only a quarter of UK adults consume the recommended dietary amount of fruit and vegetables (BHF 2018). The 'Eatwell Guide' has replaced the 'Eatwell plate' and is an excellent visual representation of the Government's dietary advice and nutrient recommendations (PHE 2018).

Sedentary lifestyle

People at high risk of, or with, CVD should do at least 150 minutes of moderate intensity aerobic activity *or* 75 minutes of vigorous intensity aerobic activity or a mix of moderate and vigorous aerobic activity weekly, in line with national guidance for the general population. If unable to do this, exercising at their maximum safe capability is advised (NICE 2014a). This may mean walking a few lengths of their hall or once around the house – any activity is beneficial. Two out of 5 adults in the UK do not achieve these recommended levels of physical activity (BHF 2018a).

Hypertension

Nearly 30 per cent of people in the UK have hypertension, and up to half are not receiving treatment. People with high blood pressure are three times more likely to develop heart disease (BHF 2018a). Using anti-hypertensive drugs to lower blood pressure is associated with reductions in CHD, stroke, heart failure and both cardiovascular and total mortality (SIGN 2017).

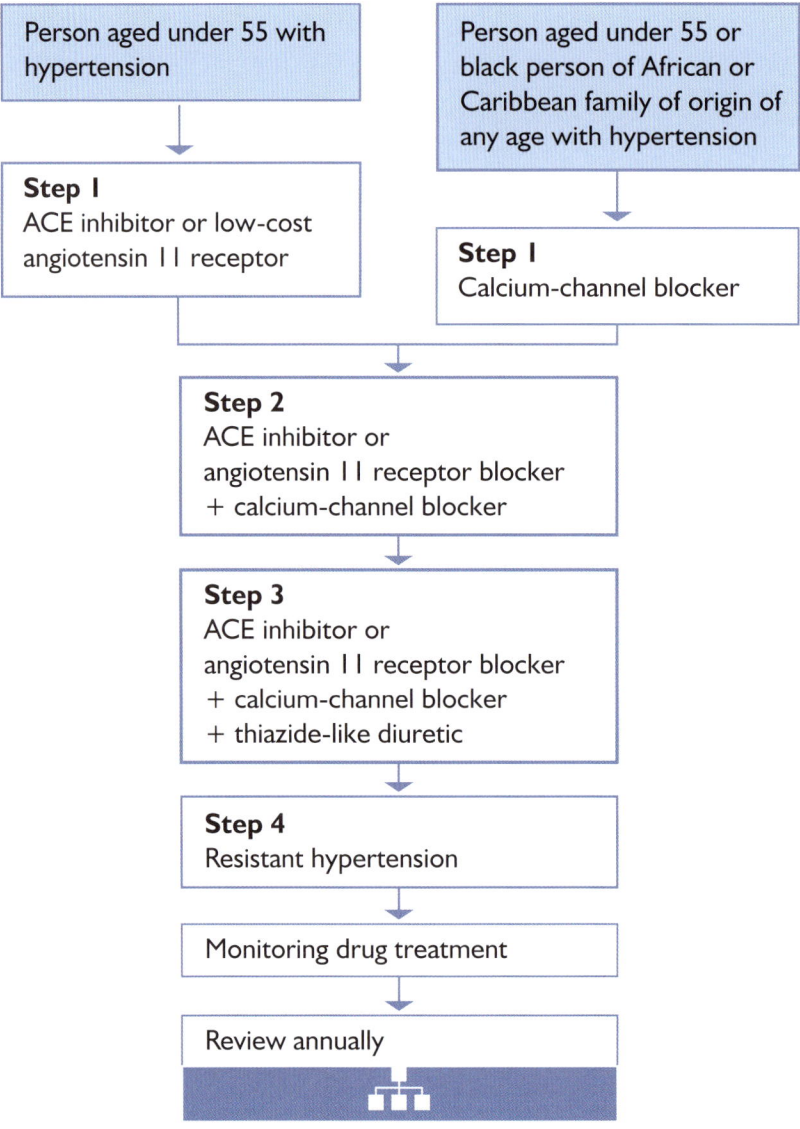

Figure 15.1: Management of hypertension

Hypertension accelerates the development and progression of atherosclerosis, and sustained elevation of BP can destabilise vascular lesions and precipitate acute coronary events. In fact, hypertension, in itself, can cause myocardial ischaemia in the absence of CHD. The CVS risks attributed to hypertension can be greatly reduced by optimal control of BP (Oladipup *et al.* 2011).

Patients with CHD, diabetes, chronic kidney disease (CKD) or established target organ damage (including heart failure, stroke, TIA, peripheral arterial disease, abnormal renal function, retinopathy or left ventricular hypertrophy), with a BP >135/85mmHg, should be offered antihypertensive therapy (SIGN 2017). JBS3 recommends a target of <140/80mmHg for isolated CHD, and <130/80mmHg if a patient has diabetes or CKD (with ACR >3mg/mmol) and <150/90 in patients over 80 years of age (JBS 2014). Treatment steps for hypertension are illustrated in Figure 15.1 (NICE 2011).

Hypercholesterolaemia

Primary prevention

Atorvastatin 20mg should be offered for the primary prevention of CVD to people who have a 10 per cent or greater 10-year risk of developing CVD. Estimate the level of risk using the QRISK3 assessment tool (NICE 2016).

Secondary prevention

If a person has established CHD, then start statin treatment with Atorvastatin 80mg, or a lower dose if any of the following apply:

- Potential drug interactions
- High risk of adverse effects
- Patient preference
- Target cholesterol level.

After 3 months of treatment, measure total cholesterol, HDL cholesterol and non-HDL cholesterol in all patients who have been started on high-intensity statin treatment. If a greater than 40 per cent reduction in non-HDL cholesterol has not been achieved:

- Discuss adherence and timing of dose
- Optimise adherence to diet and lifestyle measures
- Consider increasing dose if started on less than Atorvastatin 80mg and the person is judged to be at higher risk because of comorbidities, risk score or using clinical judgement.

Statins should be prescribed using a 'lower is better' approach to achieve values of at least <2.5mmol/l for non-HDL-C (equivalent to <1.8mmol/l for LDL-C). Recheck liver function tests (LFTs) within 3 months of starting treatment, and again at 12 months. Further monitoring is not necessary unless clinically indicated.

Smoking

More than 1 in 6 adults smoke in the UK, with 20,000 deaths from CVD attributed to smoking each year (BHF 2018a). Smoking cessation intervention by the GPN is an essential component of managing cardiovascular risk in these high-risk patients. At every opportunity, ask people if they smoke and advise them to stop smoking in a way that is sensitive to their preferences and needs (NICE 2018a). You should refer people who want to stop smoking to a local specialist stop smoking service, where expert advice on quitting aids can be discussed on an individual basis.

Alcohol

Excessive alcohol intake is a well-established risk factor for CHD and patients must be advised that even light to moderate alcohol consumption can increase risk (SIGN 2017). Binge drinking should definitely be avoided (NICE 2014a). The GPN is ideally placed to discuss the risks and work with the patient to plan how to reduce the volume of alcohol consumed, preferably establishing several drink-free days each week.

Diabetes

The importance of the association between diabetes and CHD can be illustrated by findings from the Framingham Study (Kannel & McGee 1979) and the Multiple Risk Factor Intervention Trial (MRFIT) (Stamler *et al.* 1993). The presence of diabetes doubled the age-adjusted risk for cardiovascular disease in men and tripled it in women.

A systematic review and meta-analysis have revealed that women with diabetes have more than a 40 per cent higher risk of incidence of CHD than men with diabetes (Sanne *et al.* 2014). Intensive glycaemic control has been shown to result in a 58 per cent reduction in major cardiovascular events in type 1 diabetes (UKPDS 1998).

Reducing HbA1c levels as soon as possible after diagnosis of type 2 diabetes results in a reduction in diabetes-related complications, including myo¬cardial infarction (MI) and all-cause mortality. This early reduction in the HbA1c level explains the so-called legacy effect found in the UKPDS (UKPDS 2012). This persistence in effect was seen for MI and for all-cause mortality. At the end of the original study, MI was reduced by 16 per cent with intensive HbA1c control, versus conventional control. At 10 years of follow-up, there was a 15 per cent risk reduction with intensive control.

Management of glycaemic control is an essential part of CHD management in primary care and cannot be viewed separately. Achieving and maintaining optimal glycaemic control is essential to reduce the long-term risks of diabetes.

Myocardial infarction

Following a myocardial infarction (MI), all patients must be treated with an ACE inhibitor, dual anti-platelet therapy, a statin and a beta blocker (NICE 2013). All patients (regardless of their age) should also be advised about and offered a cardiac rehabilitation programme with an exercise component (NICE 2013).

Myocardial infarction is more common in patients with diabetes than those without, and patients with diabetes are 50 per cent more likely to have a fatal MI. Studies show that good glycaemic control can positively influence the long-term development of CVD and mortality in patients with diabetes (Barnett 2010, Bergenstal 2015). Glycaemic control and management play an integral part in the management of the patient with CHD.

A vital aspect of the GPN's role is helping to increase the quality of life of the patient living with CHD. Patients require support with everything from pharmacological management to their personal, sexual and professional relationships, which can all be adversely affected by this long-term condition (Mendes 2015).

The diagnosis of MI can sometimes be underestimated by patients, especially if they have only spent one night in hospital over a weekend and have not had a chance to liaise with the Cardiac Nurse Specialist. They may not associate having a stent inserted with 'having a heart attack'. Providing them with the relevant information and health promotion advice will enable them to make positive health decisions and set realistic goals.

Atrial fibrillation

Atrial fibrillation (AF) is one of the most common forms of abnormal heart rhythm and a major cause of stroke. Nearly 1.3 million people in the UK have been diagnosed with AF and it is estimated that there are at least 500,000 people living with undiagnosed AF (BHF 2018a). Despite good progress in the management of patients with AF, it remains one of the major causes of stroke, heart failure, sudden death and cardiovascular morbidity in the world (ESC 2016a). By 2030, 14–17 million AF patients are anticipated in the European Union, with up to 215,000 newly diagnosed patients per year (Zoni-Berisso *et al.* 2014).

AF is independently associated with a two-fold increased risk of all-cause mortality in women and a 1.5-fold increase in men (Anderson *et al.* 2013). Contemporary studies show that 20–30 per cent of patients with an ischaemic stroke have AF diagnosed before, during or after the initial event (Kishore *et al.* 2014).

ECG documentation is required to establish the diagnosis of AF. A full cardiovascular history and examination is required in all patients (ESC 2016a). Renal function must be assessed to detect kidney disease and support correct dosing of oral anticoagulation therapy (ESC 2016a).

Oral anticoagulation therapy (OAC) can prevent the majority of ischaemic strokes in AF and can prolong life. It is superior to no treatment, or treatment with aspirin, with universal clinical benefit (Ruff *et al.* 2014). The introduction of the CHA2DS2-VASC score has simplified the initial decision for OAC in AF patients. (Lip *et al.* 2010). Patients with non-valvular AF, with a CHA2DS2-VASC score of 1 or more for men and 2 or more for women, should be offered anticoagulation (ESC 2016a).

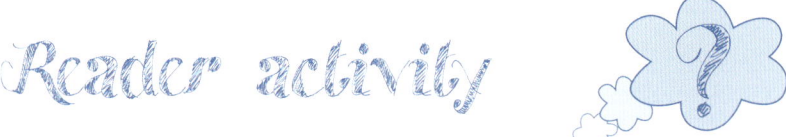

Find out what a CHA2DS2-VASC is, and discuss this with your mentor in practice.

Box 15.1: Reader activity

Several bleeding risk scores have been developed. The most common is the HAS-BLED score. A score of 3 or more indicates increased one-year bleed risk on anticoagulation sufficient to justify caution or more regular review (Pisters *et al.* 2010). A high bleeding risk score should generally not result in withholding OAC. Rather, bleeding risk factors should be identified and treatable factors corrected (ESC 2016a).

Non-vitamin K antagonist oral anticoagulants (NOACs), which include Dabigatran, Apixaban, Edoxaban and Rivaroxaban, are suitable alternatives to warfarin for stroke prevention in AF. Their use is increasing rapidly in clinical practice (Olesen *et al.* 2015).

All NOACs have a predictable effect without any need for regular anticoagulation monitoring (ESC 2016a). Antiplatelet therapy (aspirin or clopidogrel) is not recommended for stroke prevention in AF, due to poor efficacy and an increased risk of bleeding (NICE 2014b).

Referral to secondary care on diagnosis of AF is essential so that further investigations, including transthoracic echocardiography, can be performed. Decisions will be made regarding suitability for electrical cardioversion or catheter ablation where appropriate. However, anticoagulation should not be delayed, and decisions should be made to start either warfarin or NOAC after a discussion between the health care professional and the patient around the potential risks and benefits of both therapies (NICE 2014b; NICE, 2016).

Heart failure

Heart failure is a syndrome characterised by typical symptoms (breathlessness, ankle swelling and fatigue) that may be accompanied by signs (elevated jugular venous pressure, pulmonary crackles and peripheral oedema) caused by a structural and/or functional cardiac abnormality, resulting in reduced cardiac output and/or elevated intracardiac pressures at rest or during stress (ESC 2016b).

Causes and prevalence

The causes of heart failure are many, and include CHD (the most common cause), hypertension, cardiomyopathies, valvular heart disease, congenital heart disease, arrhythmias (e.g. AF), sepsis, thiamine deficiency, end-stage CKD, obesity and drugs (e.g. cocaine, alcohol or non-steroidal anti-inflammatory drugs) (Yancy *et al.* 2013).

The prevalence of heart failure slowly increases with age until about 65 years of age, and then more rapidly. In the UK the prevalence is estimated to be about:

- 1 in 35 people aged 65–74
- 1 in 15 people aged 75–84
- Just over 1 in 7 people aged 85 or older (NICE 2018a).

The European Society of Cardiology have developed terminology to classify heart failure, using preserved ejection fraction, moderate-range ejection fraction and reduced ejection fraction (ESC 2006b, table 3.1).

Table 15.2 is the New York Heart Association (NYHA) functional classification of heart failure, based on severity of symptoms and relative limitation of physical activity (Yancy *et al.* 2013).

Table 15.1: New York Heart Association (NYHA) functional classification of heart failure

Class	Patient symptoms
Class I (mild)	No limitation of physical activity. Ordinary physical activity does not cause undue fatigue, rapid/irregular heartbeat (palpitation) or shortness of breath (dyspnea).
Class II (mild)	Slight limitation of physical activity. Comfortable at rest, but ordinary physical activity results in fatigue, rapid/irregular heartbeat (palpitation) or shortness of breath (dyspnea).
Class III (moderate)	Marked limitation of physical activity. Comfortable at rest, but less than ordinary physical activity causes fatigue, rapid/irregular heartbeat (palpitation) or shortness of breath (dyspnea).
Class IV (severe)	Unable to carry out physical activity without discomfort. Symptoms of fatigue, rapid/irregular heartbeat (palpitation) or shortness of breath (dyspnea) are present at rest. If any physical activity is undertaken, discomfort increases.

Prognosis

About 50 per cent of patients with heart failure die within 5 years of diagnosis (Yancy *et al.* 2013). The most recent European data demonstrate that 12-month all-cause mortality rates for hospitalised patients were 17 per cent and 7 per cent for stable/ambulatory patients (ESC 2016b). Most deaths are due to cardiovascular causes, mainly sudden death and worsening heart failure. Over the past 30 years, improvements in treatments have improved survival rates, but the outcomes remain unsatisfactory.

Diagnosis and investigations

There is no symptom or sign that is both sensitive and specific for the diagnosis of heart failure, which makes it difficult to reach a clinical diagnosis. Patients presenting with suspected chronic heart failure should receive a range of tests, such as natriuretic peptide (B-type natriuretic peptide BNP) or NT-proBNP level. Interpretation of natriuretic peptide can be complicated, as it can be reduced by obesity, ACE inhibitors and beta blockers, and increased by hypoxia, CKD, sepsis, diabetes and female gender (NICE 2018b).

Other tests should usually include a full blood count, blood glucose, serum urea and electrolytes, thyroid function, urinalysis, ECG and chest x-ray. Echocardiography is recommended in patients with raised BNP or NT-proBNP level or an abnormal ECG, to confirm the diagnosis and establish the underlying cause (SIGN 2016).

Pulmonary function tests may be considered in patients with comorbid lung disease to assess other causes of dyspnoea (NICE 2018b, SIGN 2016).

Management of heart failure in primary care

Patients with heart failure should be advised to aim for a salt intake of less than 6g daily and avoid 'low salt' due to its high potassium content. They should weigh themselves at a set time of day (first thing in the morning, before dressing) and report a weight gain of more than 1.5–2kg in 2 days to the health care professional who is monitoring them (SIGN 2016).

Alcohol should not be taken in excess, and if the heart failure is associated with alcohol intake they should be encouraged to stop drinking completely. Smoking cessation assistance should be offered, and patients with stable heart failure (NYHA class 11–111) should be offered a moderate intensity supervised exercise programme to give improved exercise tolerance and quality of life (SIGN 2016)

Pharmacological therapies

All patients with heart failure, NYHA 11-IV should be started on beta blocker therapy as soon as their condition is stable. All patients should be given angiotensin-converting enzyme (ACE) inhibitors or given an angiotensin-receptor blocker if intolerant to ACE inhibitors (SIGN 2016). Beta blockers and ACE inhibitors have been proven to reduce mortality and morbidity in patients with heart failure (ESC 2016b).

Mineralocorticoid/aldosterone receptor antagonists (MRAs) – Spironolactone and Eperelone – are recommended in all symptomatic patients with HFrEF and LVEF <35 per cent to reduce mortality and hospitalisation (ESC 2016b).

Diuretics are recommended to reduce the signs and symptoms of congestion and have been shown to improve exercise capacity and reduce the risk of death compared with placebo (Faris *et al.* 2012).

Ivabridine is a medication used for the symptomatic management of heart-related stable chest pain and heart failure not fully managed by beta blockers. It should be given to patients with a diagnosis of heart failure with reduced ejection fraction of NYHA 11-IV, LVEF <35, who have been admitted to hospital for heart failure in the previous 12 months but have stabilised on standard therapy for at least 4 weeks. Patients must have a sinus rhythm heart rate >75 beats per minute despite maximum tolerated dose of beta blockers (SIGN 2016b).

Angiotensin receptor neprilysin inhibitors (ARNIs) are a new class of drug, with Valsartan and Sacubitril in a single pill. These drugs enhance diuresis, natriuresis and myocardial relaxation. Vasoconstriction is reduced, as well as sodium and water retention and myocardial hypertrophy (Mangiafici *et al.* 2013). They have been shown to be superior to ACE inhibitors in reducing hospitalisation, cardiovascular mortality and overall mortality (ESC 2016b, Desai *et al.* 2006). A major study into the role of ARNIs was stopped early due to the overwhelming benefit of this drug in both death reduction and hospitalisation for heart failure (McMurray *et al.* 2014).

Annual review of all patients with CHD

An annual review should be carried out for all patients who are living with a long-term condition, and the annual review of the patient with CHD is a routine element of the GPN's role. A comprehensive history is recorded, and any symptoms assessed. The GPN should ask the patient if they have any new symptoms, such as chest pain, shortness of breath, ankle swelling, dizziness, fatigue, leg swelling or leg cramps (Schilling McCann 2002).

Routine monitoring should include physical examination involving pulse and blood pressure, height and weight and relevant blood tests. A manual pulse and BP recording can pick up atrial fibrillation which could be missed with electronic monitoring, thus missing a vital stroke prevention opportunity.

Blood tests will usually measure renal function, liver function, lipid profile, thyroid function and blood glucose. The annual review is also a perfect opportunity to discuss the patient's medication and support adherence. Non-concordance with medications – for example, in heart failure – has been linked to decompensation and preventable hospital admission (Annema *et al.* 2009).

A holistic and compassionate approach will encompass physical, psychological and social issues and go a long way towards increasing the patient's confidence in coping with and managing their condition. The annual review should focus on providing the patient with information to enable them to take control of their life, rather than depending on health care professionals. For self-management to be successful, the patient must understand their condition and recognise and manage their symptoms. It is essential that the patient understands the indications, dosing and side-effects of their medication (Brake & Jones 2017). Supplementing verbal advice with written material may be necessary to ensure the patient has access to all information needed to self-manage their condition.

Depression and coronary artery disease are closely linked because coronary artery disease can cause depression, and depression is an independent risk factor for coronary artery disease and its complications. Depression may also contribute to sudden cardiac death and increase all causes of cardiac mortality, contributing to unhealthy lifestyle and poor adherence to treatment (Khawaja *et al.* 2009). It is important to screen for depression annually, and initiate treatment plans if the patient is experiencing depression. Family members could be involved in care, where appropriate.

Summary

The role and scope of nursing practice has evolved in response to the dynamic needs of individuals, communities and healthcare services. Health services are now focused on maintaining people in their communities and keeping them out of hospital where possible. Nurse-led clinics caring for patients with coronary heart disease are ideally placed to work towards this goal; the GPN is ideally placed to plan and deliver multi-focal care to CHD patients.

Resources
British Heart Foundation – living with heart failure: https://www.bhf.org.uk/informationsupport/support/practical-support/living-with-heart-failure
HeartUK – Cholesterol charity: http://heartuk.org.uk/
NHS Choices: https://www.nhs.uk/Conditions/Coronary-heart-disease/

Box 15.2: Resources

References

Anderson, T., Magnuson, A., Bryngelsson, I.L. & Frobert, O. (2013). All-cause mortality in 272,186 patients hospitalised with incident atrial fibrillation 1995-2008: a Swedish nationwide long-term case-control study. *European Heart Journal.* **34**, 1061–67.

Annema, C., Luttik, M.L. & Jaarsma, T. (2009). Reasons for readmission in heart failure: perspectives of patients, caregivers, cardiologists and heart failure nurses. *Heart and Lung.* **38**(5), 427–34.

Barnett, K. (2010) A 12-year follow-up of all-cause mortality and cardiovascular mortality in 10.432 people with newly diagnosed diabetes in Tayside, Scotland. *Diabetic Medicine.* **27**(10), 1124–29.

Bergenstal, R.R. (2015). Glycaemic variability and diabetes complications – does it matter? *Diabetes Care.* **38**(8), 1615–21.

Brake, R. & Jones, I.D. (2017). Chronic heart failure part 2: treatment and management. *Nursing Standard.* **31**(20) 53–62.

British Heart Foundation (BHF) (2018a). https://www.bhf.org.uk/what-we-do/our-research/heart-statistics/heart-statistics-publications/cardiovascular-disease-statistics-2018 (last accessed 31.1.2019).

British Heart Foundation (BHF) (2018b). *Healthy eating.* https://www.bhf.org.uk/informationsupport/support/healthy-living/healthy-eating (last accessed 31.1.2019).

Butland, B., Jebb, S., Kopelman P. *et al.* (2007). *Foresight Report: Tackling Obesities – Future Choices – Summary of key messages.* https://assets.publishing.service.gov.uk/government/uploads/system/uploads/attachment_data/file/287937/07-1184x-tackling-obesities-future-choices-report.pdf (last accessed 31.1.2019).

Cefalu, W., Kaul, S., Hertzel, C. & Gerstein, C. (2018). Cardiovascular Outcomes Trials in Type 2 Diabetes: Where do we go from here? Reflections from a Diabetes Care Editors' Expert Forum. *Diabetes Care.* **41**, 14–31.

European Society of Cardiology (ESC) (2016a). European Society of Cardiology Guidelines for the management of atrial fibrillation in collaboration with EACTS. *European Heart Journal.* **37**, 2893–962.

European Society of Cardiology (ESC) (2016b). European Society of Cardiology Guidelines for the diagnosis and treatment of acute and chronic heart failure. *European Heart Journal.* **37**, 2129–200.

Desai, A., Claggart, B., Packer, M. Zile, M. & Rouleau, J. (2006). Influence of Sacubitril/Valsartan (LCZ696) on 30-day readmission after heart failure. *Journal of the American College of Cardiology.* **68**(3), 242–48.

Faris, R.F., Purcell, H., Poole-Wilson, P.A. & Coates, A.J. (2012) Diuretics for heart failure. *Cochrane Database Systematic Review.* **2**, CD003838

Garrison, R.J. & Castelli, W.P. (1985). Weight and 30 year mortality of men in the Framingham study. *Annals of Internal Medicine.* **103**, 1006–1009.

Joint British Societies (JBS) (2014a). Joint British Societies for the prevention of cardiovascular disease (JBS3). *Heart.* **100**(2), ii1–ii67. http://www.jbs3risk.com/pages/Who_calculator_For.htm (last accessed 31.1.2019).

Joint British Societies (JBS) (2014b). *Joint British Societies for the prevention of cardiovascular disease. JBS3 Report.* http://www.jbs3risk.com/pages/report.htm (last accessed 31.1.2019).

Kannel, W.B. & McGee, D.L. (1979). Diabetes and Cardiovascular Risk Factors – the Framingham Study. *Circulation.* **59**, 8.

Khawaja, I., Westermeyer, J., Gajwani, P. & Fernstein, R. (2009) Depression and Coronary Artery Disease. *Psychiatry.* **6**(1), 38–51.

Kishore, A., Vail, A., Majid, A., Dawson, J., Tyrell, P.J. & Smith, C.J. (2014). Detection of Atrial Fibrillation after ischaemic stroke or transient ischaemic attack: a systematic review and meta-analysis. *Stroke.* **45**, 520–26.

Loades, J. (2017). Cardiovascular Disease Prevention: where are we now? *Practice Nurse.* **47**(9), 16–20.

Lip, G.Y., Nieuwlatt, R.,, Pisters, R., Lane, D.A. & Crijins, H.J. (2010). Refining clinical risk stratification for predicting stroke and thromboembolism in atrial fibrillation using a novel risk factor-based approach; the euro-heart survey on atrial fibrillation. *Chest.* **137**, 72.

Mangiafici, S., Costello-Boerrigter, L.C., Anderson, I.A., Cataliotti, A. & Burnett, J.C. (2013). Neutral endopeptidase inhibition and the natriuretic peptide system: an evolving strategy in cardiovascular therapeutics. *European Heart Journal.* **34**, 886–93.

McMurray, J., Packer, M., Akshay, S. & Desai, M. (2014). Angiotensin-Neprilysis Inhibition versus Enalopril in Heart Failure. *The New England Journal of Medicine.* **371**(11), 993–1003.

Mendes, A. (2015). Coronary Heart Disease: a self-care, communication and quality of life. *British Journal of Community Nursing.* **20**(1), 42–43.

Miller, W.R. & Rollnick, S. (2013). *Motivational Interviewing – Helping People Change.* 3rd edn. New York: Guildford Press.

NHS Digital (2018). *Statistics on Obesity, Physical Activity and Diet.* https://files.digital.nhs.uk/publication/0/0/obes-phys-acti-diet-eng-2018-rep.pdf (last accessed 31.1.2019).

NICE (2011). *Hypertension in adults: diagnosis and management.* https://www.nice.org.uk/guidance/cg127 (last accessed 31.1.2019).

NICE (2013). *Myocardial infarction: cardiac rehabilitation and prevention of further cardiovascular disease.* https://www.nice.org.uk/guidance/cg172/chapter/1-recommendations#drug-therapy-2 (last accessed 31.1.2019).

NICE (2014a). *Cardiovascular disease: risk assessment and reduction, including lipid modification.* https://www.nice.org.uk/guidance/CG181 (last accessed 31.1.2019).

NICE (2014b). *Anticoagulation to reduce stroke risk.* https://www.nice.org.uk/guidance/qs93/chapter/Quality-statement-1-Anticoagulation-to-reduce-stroke-risk (last accessed 31.1.2019).

NICE (2016). *Cardiovascular disease: risk assessment and reduction, including lipid modification.* https://www.nice.org.uk/guidance/CG181/chapter/1-Recommendations (last accessed 20.02.2019).

NICE (2018a). *NICE smoking cessation guideline.* https://www.guidelines.co.uk/smoking-cessation/nice-smoking-cessation-guideline/454141.article (last accessed 31.1.2019).

NICE (2018b). *Chronic heart failure in adults: management.* https://www.nice.org.uk/guidance/ng106 (last accessed 31.1.2019).

Nursing and Midwifery Council (2015). *The Code: Professional standards of practice and behaviour for nurses and midwives.* https://www.nmc.org.uk/code (last accessed 31.1.2019).

Oladipup, O., Ferdinand, Z., Perry, B. & Girardin, J. (2011) Management of hypertension among patients with Coronary Heart Disease. *International Journal of Hypertension* http://dx.doi.org/10.4061/2011/653903 (last accessed 31.1.2019).

Olesen, J.B., Scorensen, R., Hansen, M.L., Lamberts, M., Weeke, P. & Mikkelsen, A.P. (2015). Non-vitamin K antagonist oral anticoagulation agents in anticoagulant naïve AF patients. *Europace.* **17**, 187–93.

Pisters, R., Lane, D.A., Nieuwlatt, R., de Vos, C.B., Crijns,H.J. & Lip G.Y. (2010). A novel user-friendly score to assess 1 year risk of major bleeding in AF patients. The Euro Heart Study. *Chest.* **138** (5), 1093–100.

Public Health England (PHE) (2018). *A Quick Guide to the Government's Healthy Eating Recommendations – The Eat Well Guide.* https://assets.publishing.service.gov.uk/government/uploads/system/uploads/attachment_data/file/595133/A_quick_guide_to_govt_healthy_eating.pdf (last accessed 31.1.2019).

Quality Outcome Framework (2017). *General Practice (GP) Collections*. https://digital.nhs.uk/services/general-practice-gp-collections (last accessed 31.1.2019).

Rabkin, S.W. & Matthewson, F.A. (1977). Relation of body weight to development of ischaemic heart disease in a cohort of young North American men after 1 26 year observational period – the Manitoba Study. *American Journal of Cardiology.* **39**, 452–58.

Ruff, C.T., Guigliano, R.P., Braunwald, E., Hoffman, E.B., Deenadayalu, N. & Ezekowitz, M.D. (2014). Comparison of the efficacy and safety of new oral anticoagulants with warfarin in patients with AF: a meta-analysis of randomised trials. *Lancet.* **383**, 955–62.

Sanne, A., Peters, E., Huxley, R. & Woodward, M. (2014). Diabetes as a risk factor for incident CHD in women compared with men. *Diabetologia.* **57**(8), 1542–51.

Schilling McCann, J. (2002). *Assessment made Incredibly Easy.* 2nd edn. Pennsylvania: Springhouse.

Scottish Intercollegiate Guidelines Network (SIGN) (2016). *Management of chronic heart failure.* http://www.sign.ac.uk/assets/sign147.pdf (last accessed 31.1.2019).

Scottish Intercollegiate Guidelines Network (SIGN) (2017). *Risk assessment and the prevention of cardiovascular disease.* http://www.sign.ac.uk/assets/sign149.pdf (last accessed 31.1.2019).

Stamler, J., Vaccaro, O., Neaton, J.D. & Wentworth, D. (1993) Diabetes, other risk factors and 12 year cardiovascular mortality for men screened in the Multiple Risk Factor Intervention Trial. *Diabetes Care.* **16**, 434.

UK Prospective Diabetes Study (UKPDS) (1998). Tight blood pressure control and risk of macrovascular and microvascular complications in type 2 diabetes: UK Prospective Diabetes Study 38, *British Medical Journal.* **317**(7160), 703–13.

UK Prospective Diabetes Study (UKPDS) (2012). UK Prospective Diabetes Study Follow-up. Early HbA1C reductions linked to a decrease in M.I. and all-cause mortality. *Value-based care in metabolic health.* **1**(2).

William, R. & Rollnick, S. (2013). *Motivational Interviewing, Helping People Change (Applications of Motivational Interviewing).* New York: Guildford Press.

Yancy, C.W., Jessup, M., Bozkurk, B., Butler, J., Casey, D.E., Drazner, M.H. and Wilkoff, B.L. (2013). Guideline for the management of Heart Failure Executive Summary: A report of the American College of Cardiology Foundation/American Heart Association Task Force on Practice Guidelines (2013). *Circulation.* **128**, 1810–52.

Zoni-Berisso, M., Lercari, F., Carazza, T. & Domenicucci, S. (2014). Epidemiology of atrial fibrillation: European perspective. *Clinical Epidemiology.* **6**, 213–20.

Chapter 16

Cancer as a long-term condition

Deborah Duncan

Introduction

Historically cancer has been considered as an acute, life-limiting condition, but many types of cancer are now seen as long-term conditions (LTCs). An estimated 1.8 million people in the UK have cancer and at least one other long-term condition (DH 2012, Macmillan Cancer Support 2015a). The number of people living more than 5 years from initial diagnosis is predicted to double from decade to decade (Cancer Research UK 2015). This shift in thinking means that care must be developed to suit the cancer patient in the long term.

Research and recommendations

Effective care therefore involves defining cancer as a long-term condition within integrated care frameworks (NHS TCST 2015). It means that clinicians in primary care are educated to deliver high-quality, holistic Cancer Care Reviews. Other recommendations from the NHS Transforming Cancer Services Team (2015) included the appointment of a named Cancer GP and a named Cancer Nurse in each GP practice.

In 2011, Macmillan Cancer Support commissioned an online survey of 251 GPNs across the UK to review the types of chronic conditions they were managing. The responses showed that, although many of them were caring for patients who had cancer as an LTC, a large proportion felt that they did not have the skills and confidence to do so. Despite this, the researchers found that GPNs do communicate effectively with patients living with cancer and are in an ideal position to support patients with these conditions. They can also support them to make positive choices about exercise and lifestyle, in order to improve their overall quality of life, and make them aware of the services and resources that are available to them (Macmillan Cancer Support 2011). GPNs also have a greater insight into the ongoing needs of patients with cancer and know how to integrate their needs into existing care pathways.

Cancer Research UK (2015) recommended that all patients diagnosed with cancer should receive:

- A holistic needs assessment, which takes into account social circumstances, mental health and comorbidities
- A written individualised care and support plan at key points on their care pathway; this plan should be shared between the patient and their designated healthcare professional
- Information on the likely side effects of treatment and how best to manage them
- Information on what to do in case of recurrence or secondary cancers
- A key contact point for rapid re-entry into the healthcare system
- A treatment summary that is completed at the end of each phase of acute treatment
- Access to patient education and healthy lifestyle and physical activity resources
- Signposting for rehabilitation, work and financial support services.

Primary care is unique in its patient approach to care. Certainly, newly diagnosed patients with cancer say they want the individualised and personalised aspects of the Cancer Care Review in primary care and these aspects should not be lost (Adams *et al.* 2011).

Having cancer and another LTC

Around 70 per cent of people with a diagnosis of cancer have at least one other long-term condition (Macmillan Cancer Support 2015a) and this can affect their survival rate. Those who have an LTC in addition to a cancer diagnosis are more likely to die within seven years of diagnosis than those without a pre-existing LTC. These patients also need more psychological support and are more likely to require formal social care than people with no other LTCs (Macmillan Cancer Care Support 2015b). They not only have to undergo ongoing cancer care but also the care that is required for an additional LTC. These people have complex needs and the care they receive should reflect this.

NICE (2016) sets out the following principles that take multimorbidity into consideration. They suggest that care should focus on:

- How the person's health conditions and their treatments interact and how this affects their quality of life
- The person's individual needs and preferences for treatments, health priorities, lifestyle and goals
- The benefits and risks of following guidance on single health conditions
- Improving quality of life by reducing treatment burden, adverse events and unplanned care
- Improving coordination of care across services.

As with any LTC, there should be an individualised management plan for each patient, with goals and plans for future care. This should include advance care planning: there should be a named individual for the coordination of care, agreed timing for follow-up and information about access to urgent care (NICE 2015). The GPN should consider the person's mental health and wellbeing and how their health problems affect their quality of life. They may need help to reduce and/or combine some of their healthcare appointments, or to review their polypharmacy. Certainly, it is helpful to consider non-pharmacological treatments, such as diet, exercise programmes and psychological treatments. There are also practical issues that need to be considered, such as social support and employment guidelines.

Chronic pain and pain management

Pain is one of the most common symptoms in cancer patients and can seriously affect their quality of life. It is defined as 'an unpleasant sensory and emotional experience associated with actual or potential tissue damage or described in terms of such damage' (Merskey & Bogduk 1994). Proper pain assessment requires measuring of pain intensity, clarifying the impact of pain on the patient and establishing a partnership with the patient to explore treatment options.

The goal of pain management is to provide evidence-based assessment and treatment of the pain. This involves regular pain assessment and proper characterisation of the pain to identify underlying pathophysiology, which can influence treatment options.

The healthcare professional first needs to ask:
- Is the pain acute or chronic?
- Is it secondary to cancer, cancer treatment, other causes, or a combination?
- Is it somatic, visceral, neuropathic or mixed?
- Is there an incidental component?
- Is it breakthrough pain?

Once the pain has been thoroughly assessed, the clinician can identify the optimal pharmacological and nonpharmacological treatment options for the patient. Medication is prescribed using the WHO pain relief ladder which categorises pain intensity according to severity and recommends analgesic agents based on their strength (CKS 2006, WHO 2017).

> **The stepwise approach, using the World Health Organization analgesic ladder**
> The steps are as follows:
> - Step 1 (mild pain): non-opioid analgesic such as paracetamol and/or nonsteroidal anti-inflammatory drug
> - Step 2 (mild-to-moderate pain): weak opioid such as codeine, dihydrocodeine or tramadol (controlled drug), with or without a non-opioid analgesic
> - Step 3 (severe pain): strong opioid such as morphine, with or without a non-opioid analgesic.
>
> At any stage you may consider the addition of a non-opioid adjuvant drug. This needs to be reviewed regularly and treatment can be stepped up or down as necessary.

Box 16.1: The stepwise approach to pain relief

Cancer pain is also associated with emotional distress and can result in an increased risk of developing depression. This pain can persist even after treatment stops (Jim & Andersen 2007).

Depression and anxiety

Depression and altered mood are commonly associated with cancer and LTCs (NICE 2009) but depression is frequently underdiagnosed and undertreated in women with breast cancer (Somerset *et al.* 2004). The results were similar in patients undergoing treatment for prostate cancer (Jayadevappa *et al.* 2012) and the incidence of depression remains high in cancer survivors, after treatment has finished. In a study by Han *et al.* (2013), 44 per cent of survivors suffered from depression, and more women (49 per cent) than men (42 per cent) had high depression scores using the Beck Depression Inventory. The researchers therefore concluded that patients should be screened for depression even after the end of treatment.

Depression definitions

- Subthreshold depressive symptoms: Fewer than 5 symptoms of depression
- Mild depression: Few, if any, symptoms in excess of the 5 required to make the diagnosis, and symptoms result in only minor functional impairment
- Moderate depression: Symptoms or functional impairment are between 'mild' and 'severe'
- Severe depression: Most symptoms, and the symptoms markedly interfere with functioning. Can occur with or without psychotic symptoms.

Box 16.2 Definitions of depression (Adapted from NICE 2009)

Employment

The Equality Act defines a person as disabled if they have 'a physical or mental impairment which has a substantial and long-term adverse effect on their ability to carry out normal day-to-day activities'. Employees with a progressive condition, such as cancer, can be classed as disabled and are protected against discrimination under the Equality Act 2010 from the day they are diagnosed. They should also be offered reasonable adjustments to their post, which may include a change in working hours or additional time off to attend medical appointments.

Transition between services

Part of the GPN's role is ensuring smooth transition between different services, which helps to support people nearing the end of life and their families. This may include attending a multidisciplinary team meeting to discuss people on the palliative care register.

Advance care planning

Advance care planning is an important aspect of end of life care and involves supporting patients and their families to make decisions about their future. Under the Mental Capacity Act, patients are able to make 'advance decisions' to refuse specific treatments.

An advance decision is also known as 'an advance decision to refuse treatment' or an ADRT or a living will. It is a decision people can make to refuse a specific type of treatment at some time in the future. It lets the family, carers and health professionals know the patient's wishes about refusing treatment. The treatments the patient is deciding to refuse must all be named in the advance decision.

An advance decision is legally binding if it complies with the Mental Capacity Act, is valid and applies to the situation. It takes precedence over decisions made in the patient's best interest by other people.

Summary

End of life care is a vast topic but the most important point is that patients and their families need to feel they have some control of the situation. The GPN's chief role is therefore to ensure that they have the information they need to make decisions about their own care, feel a sense of control, and experience a 'good death'.

Resources

Legal and ethical issues: https://www.dyingmatters.org/page/legal-and-ethical-issues
Planning for future care: http://www.ncpc.org.uk/publication/planning-your-future-care
Advance decisions: https://www.nhs.uk/conditions/end-of-life-care/advance-decision-to-refuse-treatment/

Box 16.3: Resources

References

Adams, E., Boulton, M., Rose, P., *et al.* (2011). Views of cancer care reviews in primary care: a qualitative study. *The British Journal of General Practice.* **61**(585), e173–e182. doi:10.3399/bjgp11X567108

Cancer Research UK (2015). *Achieving world class cancer outcomes: A strategy for England 2015–20.* https://www.cancerresearchuk.org/sites/default/files/achieving_world-class_cancer_outcomes_-_a_strategy_for_england_2015-2020.pdf (last accessed 1.2.2019).

Clinical Knowledge Summaries (CKD) (2016). *Palliative cancer care – pain.* https://cks.nice.org.uk/palliative-cancer-care-pain#!scenario:2 (last accessed 1.2.2019).

Department of Health (DH) (2012). *Long-term Conditions Compendium of Information.* 3rd edn. https://www.gov.uk/government/news/third-edition-of-long-term-conditions-compendium-published (last accessed 1.2.2019).

Han, K. H., Hwang, I. C., Kim, S., Bae, J. M., Kim, Y. W., Ryu, K. W., *et al.* (2013). Factors associated with depression in disease-free stomach cancer survivors. *Journal of Pain and Symptom Management.* **46**(4), 511–22.

Jayadevappa, R., Malkowicz, S.B., Chhatre, S., Johnson, J.C. & Gallo, J.J. (2012). The burden of depression in prostate cancer. *Psycho-Oncology.* **21**(12), 1338–45.

Jim, S. & Andersen, B. (2007). Meaning in life mediates the relationship between social and physical functioning and distress in cancer survivors. *British Journal of Health and Psychology.* **12**(3): 363–81.

Macmillan Cancer Support (2011). *Cancer as a long-term condition: Practice nurse pilot evaluation.* https://www.macmillan.org.uk/documents/aboutus/health_professionals/primarycare/newslettermay2013/cancerasalongtermconditionfullevaluationreportfinal2.pdf (last accessed 1.2.2019).

Macmillan Cancer Support (2015a). *1.8 million people are living with cancer and another long term condition.* https://www.macmillan.org.uk/aboutus/news/latestnews/18millionpeoplearelivingwithcancerandanotherlongtermcondition.aspx (last accessed 1.2.2019).

Macmillan Cancer Support (2015b). *Hidden at home: The social care needs of people with cancer.* http://www.macmillan.org.uk/Documents/GetInvolved/Campaigns/Carers/hidden-at-home.pdf (last accessed 1.2.2019).

Merskey, H. & Bogduk, N. (eds) (1994). *Classification of Chronic Pain: Descriptions of Chronic Pain Syndromes and Definitions of Pain Terms.* 2nd edn. Seattle, Wash: IASP Press. Also available online Exit Disclaimer.

NHS Transforming Cancer Services Team (NHS TCST) (2015). *Cancer as a long- term condition. A review of Cancer Care Reviews and a proposed model for London.* https://www.myhealth.london.nhs.uk/system/files/Cancer%20Care%20Review.pdf (last accessed 1.2.2019).

NICE (2009). *Depression in adults: recognition and management.* https://www.nice.org.uk/Guidance/CG90 (last accessed 1.2.2019).

NICE (2016). *Multimorbidity: clinical assessment and management.* https://www.nice.org.uk/guidance/NG56/chapter/Recommendations#taking-account-of-multimorbidity-in-tailoring-the-approach-to-care (last accessed 1.2.2019).

NICE (2018). *Depression in adults: recognition and management.* https://www.nice.org.uk/guidance/cg90/chapter/1-Guidance#enhanced-care-for-depression (last accessed 1.2.2019).

Somerset, W., Stout, S. C., Miller, A. H. & Musselman, D. (2004). Breast cancer and depression. *Oncology (Williston Park, NY).* **18**(8), 1021–34.

World Health Organization (WHO) (2017). *WHO's cancer pain ladder for adults.* http://www.who.int/cancer/palliative/painladder/en/ (last accessed 1.2.2019).

Chapter 17

Dementia

Deborah Duncan

Introduction

Most of us know someone who has been affected by dementia. According to Health Education England, there are 850,000 people living with dementia in the UK, with numbers set to rise to over 1 million by 2025 and 2 million by 2051 (DH 2015). It is also estimated that between 75 per cent and 89 per cent of care home residents have dementia, with many remaining undiagnosed (Stewart et al. 2014). Many are diagnosed in primary care but dementia is often underdiagnosed (Connolly et al. 2011). As a GPN, you should receive training on dementia that is appropriate to your role (DH 2015).

The government's plan is to improve public awareness and understanding of dementia, including making available a personalised risk assessment calculator as part of the NHS Health Check (DH 2015). The aim is that people with dementia across the country will have equal access to diagnosis, as for other conditions (DH 2015). GPNs will play a leading role in ensuring that people with dementia have access to the care they need.

Defining dementia

Dementia is an umbrella term for a chronic progressive disorder that affects the higher cortical functions, including memory, thinking, orientation, comprehension, calculation, learning capacity, language and judgement (Breitner 2006). There are different types of dementia and they can each affect people differently, the most common form being Alzheimer's disease. Some symptoms are noticeable in the early stages (Dubois *et al.* 2010, Román *et al.* 2004) and these commonly include:

- Cognitive symptoms
- Day-to-day memory and recall
- Concentrating, planning or organising – difficulties making decisions, solving problems or carrying out a sequence of tasks
- Speech and language
- Visuospatial skills – judging distances
- Orientation – to time and place
- Mood changes.

Generally speaking, the symptoms of dementia are insidious in onset and develop slowly but steadily over several years. The progression of the disease is characterised by deterioration in cognitive function and the patient's ability to undertake the activities of daily living. Patients may also undergo behavioural changes, such as agitation, wandering and aggression and non-cognitive symptoms such as depression, delusions and hallucinations. These patients tend to have at least one other medical condition or disability as well as dementia (World Alzheimer's Report 2014).

Assessment

In 2014 the Health Innovation Network, working with nursing and care homes, community health teams and housing providers developed the DeAR-GP (Dementia Assessment and Referral Tool). This tool aims to increase identification of possible dementia and subsequent diagnosis rates. The DeAR-GP is a case-finding tool which supports care workers to identify people who are showing signs of dementia and refer them to the appropriate healthcare professional (Health Innovation Network 2017).

Initial assessment

At the initial assessment, the clinician will need to take a history which should include cognitive, behavioural and psychological symptoms and how these affect the patient's daily life. This is often done in the primary care setting and the patient may have been referred by a carer or family member. The clinician can also use a structured instrument such as the Informant Questionnaire on Cognitive Decline in the Elderly (IQCODE) or the Functional Activities Questionnaire (FAQ) to support history taking from relatives or carers (Jorm 1994, Pfeffer *et al.* 1982).

If dementia is still suspected, the following tests are recommended by NICE (2018b):

- Conduct a physical examination
- Undertake appropriate blood and urine tests to exclude reversible causes of cognitive decline
- Use cognitive testing.

A validated, brief, structured cognitive instrument should be used for cognitive testing. These can be difficult to describe – try to observe them being used in practice. Examples include (NICE 2018b):

- The 10-point cognitive screener (10-CS)
- The 6-item cognitive impairment test (6CIT)
- The 6-item screener
- The Memory Impairment Screen (MIS)
- The Mini-Cog
- Test Your Memory (TYM).

The different criteria used to guide clinical judgement when diagnosing dementia subtypes are outlined in Box 17.1 (below). These are helpful, as it is important not to rule out dementia solely because the person has a normal score on a cognitive instrument (NICE 2018b). If the differential diagnosis is dementia, the patient should then be referred to a specialist dementia diagnostic service such as a memory clinic or a community old age psychiatry service. However, if they have presented with rapidly progressive dementia, they should be referred to a neurological service with access to tests for Creutzfeldt-Jakob disease and similar conditions (NICE 2018b).

Further tests and tools are recommended to help diagnose a dementia subtype (see Box 17.1). If there is a suspicion of Alzheimer's disease or a level of diagnostic uncertainty then FDG-PET (fluorodeoxyglucose-positron emission tomography-CT), or perfusion SPECT (single-photon emission CT), can be performed. Other tests include examining cerebrospinal fluid for either total tau, or total tau and phosphorylated-tau 181, and either amyloid beta 1–42, or amyloid beta 1–42 and amyloid beta 1–40 (NICE 2018b). The other tests are outlined in Box 17.3.

The different criteria used to guide clinical judgement when diagnosing dementia subtypes
- International consensus criteria for dementia with Lewy bodies
- International FTD criteria for frontotemporal dementia (progressive non-fluent aphasia and semantic dementia)

The different criteria used to guide clinical judgement when diagnosing dementia subtypes
- International consensus criteria for dementia with Lewy bodies
- International FTD criteria for frontotemporal dementia (progressive non-fluent aphasia and semantic dementia)
- International Frontotemporal Dementia Consortium criteria for behavioural variant frontotemporal dementia
- NINDS-AIREN criteria (National Institute of Neurological Disorders and Stroke and Association Internationale pour la Recherche et l'Enseignement en Neurosciences) for vascular dementia
- NIA criteria (National Institute on Aging) for Alzheimer's disease
- Movement Disorders Society criteria for Parkinson's disease dementia
- International criteria for Creutzfeldt-Jakob disease.

Box 17.1: Criteria used when diagnosing dementia subtypes

The different types of dementia
- Vascular dementia
- Mixed dementia
- Dementia with Lewy Bodies (DLB)
- Parkinson's Disease dementia (PDD)
- Frontotemporal dementia
- Creutzfeldt-Jacob dementia (CJD)
- Huntington's Disease
- Wernicke-Korsakoff Syndrome
- Mild cognitive impairment (MCI)
- Normal pressure hydrocephalus (NPH)

Box 17.2: The different types of dementia

Additional tests for:

1. Dementia with Lewy bodies – 123I-FP-CIT SPECT or 123I-MIBG cardiac scintigraphy.

Do not rule out dementia with Lewy bodies based solely on normal results on 123I-FP-CIT SPECT or 123I-MIBG cardiac scintigraphy.

2. Frontotemporal dementia

Either have FDG-PET or perfusion SPECT. Don't rule out frontotemporal dementia based solely on the results of structural, perfusion or metabolic imaging. There may also be a genetic cause in some people.

3. Vascular dementia

If the dementia subtype is uncertain and vascular dementia is suspected, use MRI. If MRI is unavailable or contraindicated, use CT. Note: do not diagnose vascular dementia based solely on vascular lesion burden. There can also be a genetic cause for young-onset vascular dementia.

(Adapted from NICE 2018b)

Box 17.3: Additional tests for specific diagnosis

After diagnosis

Once a patient has a dementia diagnosis, the patient and their family will need support, which should include access to a memory service or equivalent hospital- or primary-care-based multidisciplinary dementia service. In Northern Ireland, the Northern Ireland Single Assessment Tool (NISAT tool) is used. This is a single assessment tool (Health and Social Care Board 2011) which helps the nurse capture all the information needed to make a person- centred assessment of the patient.

The patient should also have a single named health or social care professional who is responsible for coordinating their care, as well as support from a local service to help them develop their care plan. The specific local services available may vary in different parts of the country (see Box 17.4, below).

>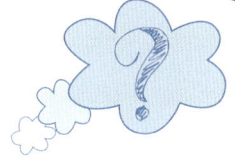
>
> ## Reader activity
>
> Find out which of the following services are available where you work:
> - Diagnostic services
> - Memory clinics
> - Third sector provision, e.g. dementia support provided by voluntary groups.
>
> Discuss this with your mentor in practice.

Box 17.4: Reader activity – dementia services

Medication

There are certain types of medication for Alzheimer's disease that can temporarily alleviate some of the symptoms or slow down their progress in some people. The two most commonly prescribed medicines for dementia are cholinesterase inhibitors and memantine (Namenda). Cholinesterase inhibitors include:

- Donepezil (Aricept)
- Galantamine (Razadyne, Razadyne ER, Reminyl)
- Rivastigmine (Exelon)

These drugs are licensed and recommended specifically for people with mild to moderate Alzheimer's and they are available in tablet, liquid or patch form.

Donepezil (Aricept, Eisai/Pfizer) is one of the AChE inhibitors used for dementia which works by increasing the concentration of acetylcholine at sites of neurotransmission. Common side effects include diarrhoea, muscle cramps, fatigue, nausea, vomiting and insomnia (NICE 2011).

Memantine (Ebixa or Axura) is a different type of medication and is recommended as an option for people with severe Alzheimer's disease, and for people with moderate Alzheimer's if cholinesterase inhibitors don't help or are not suitable. Memantine is normally given as a tablet, but it is also available as a liquid (NICE 2018a). It is a voltage-dependent, moderate-affinity, uncompetitive N-methyl-D-aspartate (NMDA) receptor antagonist that blocks the effects of glutamate which may lead to neuronal dysfunction. Side effects include dizziness, headache, constipation, somnolence and hypertension (NICE 2011).

End of life care

Dementia is a time-limiting condition, which is like a long-term condition where there is no cure. The need for palliative services depends on the individual and the type of dementia (Van der Steen *et al.* 2014). This should include advance care planning (ACP), which is considered a central component of good-quality palliative care (Detering *et al.* 2010). This is especially relevant for people with dementia, who lose the capacity to make decisions at the end of life (Vandervoort *et al.* 2014). Certainly, ACP may need to be initiated due to family involvement and patient cognitive decline (Van der Steen *et al.* 2014).

Summary

Dementia is a huge concern for the NHS; it is also a real challenge for families. This chapter has only provided a brief introduction to this topic. There are some helpful resources you can read for further information. You may also wish to register to become a Dementia Friend, in which case you will receive additional training to help you support patients and their families (see Box 17.5 below). This is an initiative established by the Alzheimer's Society. They provide Friends' Information Sessions, which are run by Dementia Friends Champions, who help people to understand what it's like to live with dementia. You can also become a Dementia Friends Champion.

Resources

DeAR-GP (Dementia Assessment Referral to GP): https://www.dear-gp.org/
Dementia Friends: https://www.dementiafriends.org.uk/
Dementia Roadmap: https://dementiaroadmap.info/
eLearning for Tier One Dementia training: https://www.e-lfh.org.uk/programmes/dementia/

Box 17.5: Resources

References

Breitner, J.C. (2006). Dementia—epidemiological considerations, nomenclature, and a tacit consensus definition. *Journal of Geriatric Psychiatry and Neurology.* **19**(3), 129–36.

Connolly, A., Gaehl, E., Martin, H., Morris, J. & Purandare, N. (2011). Underdiagnosis of dementia in primary care: variations in the observed prevalence and comparisons to the expected prevalence. *Aging and Mental Health.* **15**(8), 978–84.

Detering, K.M., Hancock, A.D., Reade, M.C. & Silvester, W. (2010) The impact of advance care planning on end of life care in elderly patients: randomised controlled trial. *British Medical Journal.* **340**, c1345.

Department of Health (DH). (2015). *Prime Minister's challenge on dementia 2020.* https://www.gov.uk/government/publications/prime-ministers-challenge-on-dementia-2020/prime-ministers-challenge-on-dementia-2020#fn:5 (last accessed 2.2.2019).

Dubois, B., Feldman, H.H., Jacova, C., *et al.* (2010). Revising the definition of Alzheimer's disease: a new lexicon. *The Lancet Neurology.* **9**(11), 1118–27.

Health Innovation Network (2017). *Dementia Assessment Referral to GP (DeAR-GP).* https://www.nice.org.uk/sharedlearning/dementia-assessment-referral-to-gp-dear-gp (last accessed 2.2.2019).

Health and Social Care Board (2011). *Northern Ireland Single Assessment Tool and Guidance.* https://www.health-ni.gov.uk/publications/northern-ireland-single-assessment-tool-and-guidance (last accessed 2.2.2019).

Jorm, A (1994). *Short Form of the Informant Questionnaire on Cognitive Decline in the Elderly (Short IQCODE).* Centre for Mental Health Research The Australian National University Canberra, Australia. https://www.alz.org/media/Documents/short-form-informant-questionnaire-decline.pdf (last accessed 20.02.2019)

NICE (2011). *Donepezil, galantamine, rivastigmine and memantine for the treatment of Alzheimer's disease.* https://www.nice.org.uk/guidance/ta217/chapter/3-The-technologies (last accessed 2.2.2019).

NICE (2018a). *Memantine Hydrochloride.* https://bnf.nice.org.uk/drug/memantine-hydrochloride.html (last accessed 2.2.2019).

NICE (2018b). *Dementia: assessment, management and support for people living with dementia and their carers.* https://www.nice.org.uk/guidance/ng97/chapter/Recommendations#diagnosis (last accessed 2.2.2019).

Pfeffer, R.I., Kurosaki, T.T., Harrah, C.H. Jr., Chance, J.M., & Filos, S. (1982). Measurement of functional activities in older adults in the community. *Journal of Gerontology.* **37**(3), 323–29.

Román, G.C., Sachdev, P., Royall, D.R., Bullock, R.A., Orgogozo, J.M., *et al.* (2004). Vascular cognitive disorder: a new diagnostic category updating vascular cognitive impairment and vascular dementia. *Journal of the Neurological Sciences.* **226**(1–2), 81–87.

Stewart, R., Hotopf, M., Dewey, M., Ballard, C., Bisla, J., *et al.* (2014). Current prevalence of dementia, depression and behavioural problems in the older adult care home sector: The South East London Care Home Survey. *Age and Ageing.* **43**(4), 562–67.

van der Steen, J.T., Radbruch, L., Hertogh, C.M., de Boer, M.E., *et al.* (2014). White paper defining optimal palliative care in older people with dementia: a Delphi study and recommendations from the European Association for Palliative Care. *Palliative Medicine.* **28**(3), 197–209.

Vandervoort, A., Houttekier, D., Vander Stichele, R., Van der Steen, J.T., & Van den Block, L. (2014). Quality of dying in nursing home residents dying with dementia: does advanced care planning matter? A nationwide postmortem study. *PloS One.* **9**(3), e91130.

World Alzheimer's Report 2014: Dementia and Risk Reduction – an analysis of protective and modifiable factors, Alzheimer's Disease International, London, September 2014.

Chapter 18

Mental illness as a long-term condition

Deborah Duncan

Introduction

The term 'mental illness' covers a wide range of mental health conditions that affect a patient's mood, thinking and behaviour. MHA (2018) suggest that there are more than 200 classified forms of mental illness. The most commonly known ones are anxiety and depression, bipolar disorder, dementia and schizophrenia. However, there are many other mental illnesses in addition to these (see Box 18.2). Mental ill health is also seen to be the largest single cause of disability in the UK, costing the economy at least £105 billion each year (Knapp et al. 2011). The cost of mental illness is also increasing (Zechmeister et al. 2008).

Mental illness in primary care

As nurses, we have historically cared for the whole person – body, soul and mind – yet in a 2012 study of the role of primary care in service provision for people with severe mental illness in the United Kingdom only 18 per cent of practice nurses reported that they had been given some form of mental health training (Reilly et al. 2012). This is an even more challenging situation when we consider just how widespread mental illness is – with 1 in 4 adults experiencing at least one diagnosable mental health problem per year and 1 in 5 older people in the community affected by depression (NHS England 2016).

Moran et al. (2000) found that there is a high prevalence of personality disorders among primary care attenders which represents a significant burden in primary care. Primary care plays a key role in the care of people with serious mental illness (NHS England 2016, Reilly *et al.*). However, many of the health professionals involved feel that caring for people with serious mental illness is too specialised for primary care (Lester *et al.* 2005). The challenge for the GPN is to help patients access the healthcare they need, which can support them with their long-term condition.

Effects of mental illness

Severe mental illness (such as bipolar disorder, schizophrenia or other psychoses) can have a massive impact on patients (Reilly *et al.* 2012). Although some people do recover, many develop long-term conditions that have to be managed (Harrison *et al.* 2001). Certainly, severe mental illness is serious and potentially life-changing (NHS England 2016, Reilly *et al.* 2012). Patients with these illnesses are also more likely to have poorer physical health than the general population (Brown 1997, Osborn *et al.* 2007, Sokal *et al.* 2004).

There are higher levels of morbidity and mortality in all age groups for those who have a serious mental illness such as schizophrenia, schizoaffective disorder, bipolar disorder or enduring depression (Osborn *et al.* 2008, Piatt *et al.* 2010, Saha *et al.* 2007). Many of the associated health problems are related to higher risks of smoking and obesity (Tamakoshi *et al.* 2010). Patients with mental illnesses are twice as likely to smoke tobacco as the general population (el-Guebaly *et al.* 2002) and smoking rates are exceptionally high among these individuals (Ziedonis *et al.* 2008).

Incidence of mental illness and attitudes to it

The number of women with mental illness is increasing, although men are more likely to commit suicide (McManus *et al.* 2016). There are about 6,000 suicides in the UK each year and suicide is the biggest killer of men up to the age of 49 (Bromley *et al.* 2014). There has also been a rise in the numbers of younger people who experience serious mental illness, with associated morbidity and mortality (Chang *et al.* 2011).

Although the incidence of mental illness is rising, the public's knowledge of mental disorders is poor and there is still a stigma surrounding the whole subject (Jorm 2000). This 'culture of suspicion' in one important reason why mental health needs often remain unaddressed (Rehm & Franck 2000). People with mental illness are doubly challenged as they have to cope with the symptoms and disabilities resulting from the disease as well as the stereotypes that arise from misconceptions about mental illness (Corrigan & Watson 2002). Improving public mental health literacy is essential in order to improve the public's acceptance of evidence-based mental healthcare (Jorm 2000).

Reader activity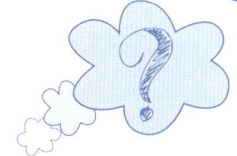

- Try to list as many forms of mental illness you can.
- Try to summarise what they are.
- What are the main methods of treatment?

Medicines used in Mental Health (NHS Scotland 2017) is a helpful document: http://www.isdscotland.org/Health-Topics/Prescribing-and-Medicines/Publications/2017-10-10/2017-10-10-PrescribingMentalHealth-Report.pdf

Also review the relevant sections in the British National Formulary (BNF) on the NICE website:

- Antidepressants: https://bnf.nice.org.uk/treatment-summary antidepressant-drugs.html
- Psychoses and associated disorders: https://bnf.nice.org.uk treatment-summary/psychoses-and-related-disorders.html

Box 18.1: Reader activity – mental illness

Mental illness in children and adolescents

Half of all mental health problems are diagnosed by the age of 14 (NHS England 2016). Amongst 5- to 19-year-olds, 1 in 8 have a mental illness (NHS Digital 2017). Despite these dramatic figures, most children and young people get no support and the average wait for routine appointments for psychological therapy was 32 weeks in 2015/16 (NHS England, 2016). The most common mental health problems in children and young people are depression, anxiety and conduct disorder (Patel *et al.* 2007).

Different types of mental illness
- Anxiety and panic attacks
- Bipolar disorder
- Body dysmorphic disorder (BDD)
- Borderline personality disorder (BPD)
- Depression

- Dissociative disorders
- Eating problems
- Hoarding
- Hypomania and mania
- Obsessive-compulsive disorder (OCD)
- Panic attacks
- Paranoia
- Personality disorders
- Phobias
- Postnatal depression & perinatal mental health
- Post-traumatic stress disorder (PTSD)
- Premenstrual dysphoric disorder (PMDD)
- Psychosis
- Schizoaffective disorder
- Schizophrenia
- Seasonal affective disorder (SAD)
- Self-harm
- Sleep problems

Box 18.2: Different types of mental illness

Prevention of mental illness

Prevention is just as important in mental illness as it is in physical illness. Certainly, Public Health England (PHE 2016) aim to 'support local areas to take positive and much needed action to improve public mental health and prevent mental health problems'. In the USA their public health action plan integrates mental health promotion and mental illness prevention with chronic disease prevention (Centers for Disease Control and Prevention 2011).

There is already evidence that lifestyle modification can improve chronic disease outcomes. For example, depressed patients appear to benefit from physical exercise as much as from psychotherapeutic interventions (Richardson *et al.* 2005).

The Five Year Forward View for Mental Health report, published in 2016, states: 'The NHS needs a far more proactive and preventative approach to reduce the long-term impact for people experiencing mental health problems and for their families, and to reduce costs for the NHS and emergency services' (NHS England 2016).

Dealing with relapse and exacerbation

GPNs also need to support clients to help them recognise the early signs of relapse or exacerbation. This is particularly important for those living with multiple disorders as they are most prone to relapse (Drake *et al.* 2005, Lam *et al.* 2000). Risk factors include increased social pressures, living in high-risk neighbourhoods and lack of dual diagnosis treatments especially for mental illness and substance or alcohol abuse (Drake *et al.* 2005, Xie *et al.* 2005). The aim should be to support patients in developing healthy, protective communities where friends can help them through their illness.

Patients with mental illness find that their health improves when they are empowered to self-care or are involved in shared decision making (Corrigan 2002). Their treatment plans should always be collaborative rather than based on a unilateral decision-making process by healthcare professionals (Corrigan 2002).

Summary

This chapter is only a brief introduction to mental illness. Nurses can help promote health and wellbeing, as well as helping to educate the general public in order to reduce social stigma for these patients. Although many patients with mental health problems are managed in secondary care as a patient group, they are more likely to have physical disorders (De Hert *et al.* 2011). The GPN is in an ideal position to help educate them about lifestyle, including smoking, diet and exercise.

Resources

1. **How to access mental health services:** https://www.nhs.uk/using-the-nhs/nhs-services/mental-health-services/how-to-access-mental-health-services/
2. **Mental Health Foundation:** https://www.mentalhealth.org.uk/a-to-z/c/children-and-young-people
3. **MIND website with helpful information about the different conditions:** https://www.mind.org.uk/information-support/types-of-mental-health-problems/
4. **Resources from the Mental Health Foundation:** https://www.mentalhealth.org.uk/projects/right-here/resources
5. **Resources from Together UK:** http://www.together-uk.org/mental-health-resources/

Box 18.3: Resources

References

Bromley, C., *et al.* (2014). *The Scottish Health Survey.* 2013 edition, volume 1, main report. [online] Edinburgh: The Scottish Government. http://www.gov.scot/Resource/0046/00464858.pdf (last accessed 2.2.2019).

Brown, S. (1997). Excess mortality of schizophrenia: a meta-analysis. *The British Journal of Psychiatry.* **171**(6), 502–508.

Chang, C.K., Hayes, R.D., Perera, G., Broadbent, M.T., Fernandes, A.C., Lee, W.E., *et al.* (2011). Life expectancy at birth for people with serious mental illness and other major disorders from a secondary mental health care case register in London. *PloS One.* **6**(5), e19590.

Centers for Disease Control and Prevention (2011). *Public Health Action Plan to Integrate Mental Health Promotion and Mental Illness Prevention with Chronic Disease Prevention.* http://www.mhrb.org/dbfiles/docs/Brochure/11_220990_Sturgis_MHMIActionPlan_FINAL-Web_tag508.pdf (last accessed 2.2.2019).

Corrigan, P.W. & Watson, A.C. (2002). Understanding the impact of stigma on people with mental illness. *World Psychiatry.* **1**(1), 16.

De Hert, M., Cohen, D., Bobes, J., Cetkovich-Bakmas, M., Leucht, S., Ndetei, D.M., Newcomer, J.W., Uwakwe, R., Asai, I., Möller, H.J., Gautam, S., *et al.* (2011). Physical illness in patients with severe mental disorders. II. Barriers to care, monitoring and treatment guidelines, plus recommendations at the system and individual level. *World Psychiatry: Official Journal of the World Psychiatric Association (WPA).* **10**(2), 138–51.

Drake, R.E., Wallach, M.A. & McGovern, M.P. (2005). Special section on relapse prevention: Future directions in preventing relapse to substance abuse among clients with severe mental illnesses. *Psychiatric Services.* **56**(10), 1297–1302. Atlanta: US Department of Health and Human Services.

el-Guebaly, N., Cathcart, J., Currie, S., Brown, D. & Gloster, S. (2002). Smoking cessation approaches for persons with mental illness or addictive disorders. *Psychiatric Services.* **53**(9), 1166–70.

Gene-Cos, N. (2006). Post-Traumatic Stress Disorder: The Management of PTSD in Adults and Children in Primary and Secondary Care. National Collaborating Centre for Mental Health. London & Leicester: Gaskell & The British Psychological Society. *Psychiatric Bulletin.* **30**(9), 357.

Harrison, G., Hopper, K., Craig, T., Laska, E., Siegel, C., *et al.* (2001). Recovery from psychotic illness: a 15- and 25-year international follow-up study. *British Journal of Psychiatry.* **178**, 506–17.

Jorm, A.F. (2000). Mental health literacy: Public knowledge and beliefs about mental disorders. *British Journal of Psychiatry.* **177**(5), 396–401.

Knapp, M., McDaid, D. & Parsonage, M. (2011). *Mental health promotion and mental illness prevention: The economic case.* http://eprints.lse.ac.uk/39300/1/Mental_health_promotion_and_mental_illness_prevention(author).pdf (last accessed 2.2.2019).

Lam, D.H., Bright, J., Jones, S., Hayward, P., Schuck, N., Chisholm, D. & Sham, P. (2000). Cognitive therapy for bipolar illness—a pilot study of relapse prevention. *Cognitive Therapy and Research.* **24**(5), 503–20.

Lester, H., Tritter, J.Q. & Sorohan, H. (2005). Patients' and health professionals' views on primary care for people with serious mental illness: focus group study. *British Medical Journal.* **330**(7500), 1122.

McManus, S., Bebbington, P., Jenkins, R. & Brugha T. (eds.) (2016). *Mental health and wellbeing in England: Adult Psychiatric Morbidity Survey 2014.* Leeds: NHS Digital. http://content.digital.nhs.uk/catalogue/PUB21748/apms-2014-full-rpt.pdf (last accessed 2.2.2019).

Mental Health America (MHA) (2018). *Mental Illness and the Family: Recognizing Warning Signs and How to Cope.* https://www.mentalhealthamerica.net/recognizing-warning-signs (last accessed 2.2.2019).

Moran, P., Jenkins, R., Tylee, A., Blizard, R. & Mann, A. (2000). The prevalence of personality disorder among UK primary care attenders. *Acta Psychiatrica Scandinavica.* **102**(1), 52–57.

NHS Digital (2017). *Mental Health of Children and Young People in England, 2017.* https://files.digital.nhs.uk/F6/A5706C/MHCYP%202017%20Summary.pdf (last accessed 2.2.2019).

NHS England (2016). *The Five Year Forward View for Mental Health.* https://www.england.nhs.uk/wp-content/uploads/2016/02/Mental-Health-Taskforce-FYFV-final.pdf (last accessed 2.2.2019).

NHS Scotland (2017). *Medicines Used in Mental Health. Years 2006/07 to 2016/17.* http://www.isdscotland.org/Health-Topics/Prescribing-and-Medicines/Publications/2017-10-10/2017-10-10-PrescribingMentalHealth-Report.pdf (last accessed 2.2.2019).

Osborn, D.P., Levy, G., Nazareth, I., Petersen, I., Islam, A. & King, M.B. (2007). Relative risk of cardiovascular and cancer mortality in people with severe mental illness from the United Kingdom's General Practice Research Database. *Archives of General Psychiatry.* **64**(2), 242–49.

Osborn, D., Levy, G., Nazareth, I. & King, M. (2008). Suicide and severe mental illnesses. Cohort study within the UK general practice research database. *Schizophrenia Research.* **99**, 134–138.

Patel, V., Flisher, A.J., Hetrick, S. & McGorry, P. (2007). Mental health of young people: a global public-health challenge. *The Lancet.* **369**(9569), 1302–313.

Piatt, E.E., Munetz, M.R. & Ritter, C. (2010). An examination of premature mortality among decedents with serious mental illness and those in the general population. *Psychiatric Services.* **61**, 663–68.

Public Health England (PHE) (2016). *Improving the mental health of children and young people.* https://www.gov.uk/government/publications/improving-the-mental-health-of-children-and-young-people (last accessed 20.2.2019).

Rehm, R.S. & Franck, L.S. (2000). Long-term goals and normalization strategies of children and families affected by HIV/AIDS. *Advances in Nursing Science.* **23**, 69–82.

Reilly, S., Planner, C., Hann, M., Reeves, D., Nazareth, I. & Lester, H. (2012). The role of primary care in service provision for people with severe mental illness in the United Kingdom. *PloS One.* **7**(5), e36468.

Richardson, C.R., Faulkner, G., McDevitt, J., Skrinar, G.S., Hutchinson, D.S. & Piette, J.D. (2005). Integrating physical activity into mental health services for persons with serious mental illness. *Psychiatric Services.* **56**(3), 324–31.

Saha, S., Chant, D. & McGrath, J. (2007). A systematic review of mortality in schizophrenia: is the differential mortality gap worsening over time? *Archives of General Psychiatry.* **64**, 1123–31.

Sokal, J., Messias, E., Dickerson, F. B., Kreyenbuhl, J., Brown, C. H., Goldberg, R.W. & Dixon, L.B. (2004). Comorbidity of medical illnesses among adults with serious mental illness who are receiving community psychiatric services. *The Journal of Nervous and Mental Disease.* **192**(6), 421–27.

Tamakoshi, A., Kawado, M., Ozasa, K., Tamakoshi, K., Lin, Y., et al. (2010). Impact of smoking and other lifestyle factors on life expectancy among Japanese: findings from the Japan Collaborative Cohort (JACC) Study. *Journal of Epidemiology.* **20**, 370–76.

Xie, H., McHugo, G. J., Fox, M. B. & Drake, R. E. (2005). Special section on relapse prevention: Substance abuse relapse in a ten-year prospective follow-up of clients with mental and substance use disorders. *Psychiatric Services.* **56**(10), 1282–87.

Zechmeister, I., Kilian, R. & McDaid, D. (2008). Is it worth investing in mental health promotion and prevention of mental illness? A systematic review of the evidence from economic evaluations. *BMC Public Health.* **8**(1), 20.

Ziedonis, D., Hitsman, B., Beckham, J.C., Zvolensky, M., Adler, L.E., Audrain-McGovern, et al. (2008). *Tobacco use and cessation in psychiatric disorders: National Institute of Mental Health report.*

Chapter 19

Conclusion

Deborah Duncan

Introduction

This book is about the foundations of general practice nursing and this chapter is about the extra things you need to know but of course it doesn't include everything! We are all constantly learning and updating our knowledge and skills. As healthcare professionals, we each have particular knowledge and skills and we may be working in diverse contexts with different levels of autonomy and responsibility. We are, however, accountable for our own work and should exercise professional judgement in our own roles (NMC 2015). We need to be aware of the limits of our own competency and uphold the *Code* (NMC 2015).

Following the NMC Code

The NMC Code has four key standards that we are expected to follow no matter where we work and what role we have:

1. Prioritise people
2. Practise effectively
3. Preserve safety
4. Promote professionalism and trust.

Prioritise people

One key principle of the NMC Code (2015) is that we put the interests of our patients first. Their care and safety are our main concern. We also need to ensure that we maintain their dignity, treat them with respect and uphold their rights. This means working in partnership with patients to ensure that we consider their worries and concerns and respect the contribution that they can make to their own health and wellbeing. These are the underpinning principles of self-management and the expert patient programmes.

Practise effectively

Another key aspect of the Code is that we practise effectively, ensuring that we 'assess need and deliver or advise on treatment or give help (including preventative or rehabilitative care) without too much delay, to the best of [our] abilities, on the basis of best available evidence' (NMC 2015, p. 9).

As nurses, we need to deliver evidence-based nursing and reflect on our own practice, as this will help us identify areas for improvement (RCN 2018). Evidence-based nursing is similar to evidence-based medicine, in that it requires 'the conscientious, explicit, and judicious use of current best evidence in making decisions about the care of individual patients' (Sackett *et al.* 1996). It is a directive approach to nursing care, which is based upon personal clinical expertise, in combination with the most current, relevant research available in the area (Melnyk 2011).

As part of our revalidation as nurses, we also need to record a minimum of five written reflections on our own continuing professional development and/or practice-related events over the three years.

Preserve safety

In addition, we have to ensure that we deliver effective and safe care. Again, a key aspect of this is ensuring that we work within the limits of our competence. We are expected to exercise a professional 'duty of candour' and raise concerns immediately whenever we see patients or public safety being put at risk. A key part of this involves dealing with medication issues in general practice and this subject is covered below.

Promote professionalism and trust

The fourth standard of the NMC Code (2015) is that, as nurses, we are always expected to uphold the reputation of the profession. In other words, at an individual level we should uphold the standards of practice and behaviour set out in the Code. In general practice this means that every GPN should be 'a model of integrity and leadership for others to aspire to' (NMC 2015, p. 17), understanding the history and background of our specific profession and being a model general practice nurse to the other 1000 nurses working in general practice (QNI 2015). Certainly, we all need to be aware of the fact that 'there is much that needs to change to both plan for the next generation of nurses and to support those who make up the current workforce in primary care' (QNI 2015, p. 32).

Medication issues

It's important to bear in mind that:
- A quarter of the population have a long-term condition
- A quarter of people over 60 have two or more long-term conditions
- With an ageing population, the use of polypharmacy is increasing.

Despite these facts, between 30 and 50 per cent of medicines prescribed for long-term conditions are not taken as intended (NICE 2016). One way to ensure that this situation improves is to ensure that any decisions about medicines are made jointly between the person taking the medicine and the prescriber. In general practice we may be working under a patient specific direction (PSD) or a patient group direction (PGD). Either way, we must ensure that patients are provided with enough information to make informed choices (NICE 2016). For instance, in general practice a GPN may carry out a travel health consultation about antimalarials with a patient who is travelling to Africa.

Medication reviews

All patients who are prescribed medications are invited to a structured medication review (NICE 2016). The purpose of this review is to optimise the use of medicines, identify medicines that could be stopped or need a dosage change, or recognise when new medicines that are needed. In many Trusts and GP surgeries, a community pharmacist will carry out these reviews as they are well placed to identify and resolve pharmaceutical care issues and improve healthcare (Krska *et al.* 2001). Certainly, community pharmacists can provide effective support for patients in nursing homes as they can review their medication and make recommendations, sometimes leading to a substantial change in patients' medication regimens without any change in drug costs (Zermansky *et al.* 2006).

There are various methods whereby medications can be supplied and administered (NMC 2009):

- Patient specific direction (PSD)
- Patient medicines administration chart (medicines administration record MAR)
- Patient group direction (PGD)
- Medicines Act exemption
- Standing order
- Homely remedy protocol
- Prescription forms (FP10).

Patient group directions

Often in primary care, we administer medication (such as a flu vaccine) under a patient group direction (PGD). This is a written instruction that allows listed healthcare professionals to administer named medicines in an identified clinical situation. It removes the need for an individual patient-specific prescription from an approved prescriber. The Human Medicines Regulations (2012) require that a PGD must be signed by a pharmacist.

The PGD must include:

- The period during which the PGD is to have effect
- The description or class of medicinal product
- The clinical situations in which it is to be used
- The clinical criteria under which a person is to be eligible for treatment
- A statement about any class of person to be excluded
- The circumstances in which further advice should be sought from a doctor or dentist
- The pharmaceutical form or forms in which the medicinal products of that description or class are to be administered
- The strength or maximum strength, the applicable dosage or maximum dosage, the route and frequency of administration and the minimum or maximum period of administration
- Any relevant warnings
- The circumstances in which any follow-up action will be needed
- The records should include the supply, or the administration, of products.

There are examples of PGDS for immunisations on the Public Health England (PHE) website: https://www.gov.uk/government/collections/immunisation-patient-group-direction-pgd

In practice all PGDs should be signed by a doctor, the head of the nursing team and a community pharmacist.

Reader activity

Please review the PGDs in your area of practice. You will need to sign one for each medication you administer unless there is a PSD.

Box 19.1: Reader activity – patient group directions

Patient specific directions

A patient specific direction (PSD) is a written instruction from a qualified prescriber for a specific medication. Each individual patient must have a separate form. The PSD includes the name of the medication, dose, route, frequency and form of delivery. The instructions must also include the patient's name, date of birth and address. This is not a prescription but a direction to administer medication and it must be signed by a registered prescriber. It authorises the delegated person to administer medication on the prescriber's behalf (NMC 2009). If there is a PSD, there is no need for a PGD.

Consent

Consent is something that you will have considered in detail during your general nurse training so this should just be a refresher. It is about consenting to treatment and refers to the principle that a person must give permission before they receive any type of treatment or test. The clinician must provide an explanation of what is being done. The principle of consent is also an important part of medical ethics and takes into consideration international human rights law. For consent to be valid, it must be voluntary and informed, and the person consenting must have the mental capacity to make the decision.

- Voluntary – the decision to consent or not to consent to treatment must be made by the person themselves. It must not be influenced by medical staff, friends or family.
- Informed – the person must be given all the information they need about the treatment, including the benefits and risks and whether there are alternative treatments. This also includes information about what will happen if the treatment doesn't go ahead.
- Capacity – the person must be capable of giving consent. This means they understand the information and can make an informed decision.

Sometimes patients don't have the capacity to decide about their treatment. They may have appointed a lasting power of attorney (LPA). The clinician treating them can give treatment if they believe it's in the person's best interests. There are also some exceptions when treatment may be able to go ahead without the person's consent – for instance, when someone requires emergency treatment to save their life.

> **Resources**
>
> For additional resources you can utilise medicines management standards but in 2019 the NMC have stopped using national standards. Please also refer to your local standards.
> https://www.nmc.org.uk/standards/standards-for-post-registration/standards-for-medicines-management/

Box 19.2: Resources

References

Gov.uk (2012). *The Human Medicines Regulations 2012.* http://www.legislation.gov.uk/uksi/2012/1916/contents/made (last accessed 3.2.2019).

Krska, J., Cromarty, J. A., Arris, F., Jamieson, D., Hansford, D., *et al.* (2001). Pharmacist-led medication review in patients over 65: a randomized, controlled trial in primary care. *Age and Ageing.* **30**(3), 205–11.

Melnyk, B.M. (2011). *Evidence-based practice in nursing & healthcare: A guide to best practice.* Philadelphia, PA: Lippincott Williams & Wilkins. pp. 3–7. ISBN 978-1-60547-778-7.

NICE (2016). *Medicines optimisation.* https://www.nice.org.uk/guidance/qs120 (last accessed 3.2.2019).

NMC (2009). *Standards for medicines management.* https://www.nmc.org.uk/standards/standards-for-post-registration/standards-for-medicines-management/ (last accessed 3.2.2019).

NMC (2015). *The Code.* https://www.nmc.org.uk/globalassets/sitedocuments/nmc-publications/nmc-code.pdf (last accessed 3.2.2019).

Queen's Nursing Institute (QNI) (2015). *General Practice Nursing. A Time of Opportunity in the 21st Century.* https://www.qni.org.uk/wp-content/uploads/2016/09/gpn_c21_report.pdf (last accessed 3.2.2019).

Royal College of Nursing (RCN) (2018). *Revalidation requirements: Reflection and reflective discussion.* https://www.rcn.org.uk/professional-development/revalidation/reflection-and-reflective-discussion (last accessed 3.2.2019).

Sackett, D., Rosenberg, W., Gray, J., Hayes, R. & Richardson, W. (1996). Evidence based medicine: what it is and what it isn't. *British Medical Journal.* 312.

Zermansky, A.G., Alldred, D.P., Petty, D.R., Raynor, D.K., Freemantle, N., Eastaugh, J. & Bowie, P. (2006). Clinical medication review by a pharmacist of elderly people living in care homes—randomised controlled trial. *Age and Ageing.* **35**(6), 586–91.

Index

action plan *100, 101*
advance care planning *177, 187*
alcohol consumption *162*
alpha-1 antitrypsin (A1AT) deficiency *135*
Alzheimer's disease *183*
Alzheimer's disease medication *186*
anaphylaxis *65*
anti-malarial medication *72, 73, 74*
anxiety *176*
asthma *137–141*
asthma diagnosis *137–140*
asthma-COPD overlap syndrome (ACOS) *134*
atherosclerosis *123*
atrial fibrillation (AF) *163*

benign prostatic hyperplasia (BPH) *46*
blood pressure control in diabetes *114, 118*
breast awareness *41*
breast cancer risk factors *40*
breast cancer screening *40*
breathlessness *140*
bronchodilator reversibility (BDR) *138*
bronchodilators *142*

Calgary-Cambridge model *13*
call and recall system *30*
cancer *40, 173–178*
cancer and employment *177*
cardiovascular risk *157, 158*
care plan *100*
cervical cancer, epidemiology *28*
cervical cytology *27–33*

cervical screening *27*
cervical screening, eligibility *30*
cervical screening, intervals by age *29*
Charcot foot *124*
chikungunya *71*
cholesterol in diabetes *114, 118*
chronic kidney disease (see also CKD) *151–155*
chronic obstructive pulmonary disease (see also COPD) *134, 140*
chronic pain *175*
CKD diagnosis *152*
CKD management *154*
CKD screening *152*
Clinical Commissioning Groups (CCGs) *4*
cognitive testing *183*
communication *12*
consent *201*
consultation, aims of *13*
consultation skills *11–15*
contraception *37–39*
COPD diagnosis *134, 135*
coronary heart disease (CHD) *157–168*
coronary heart disease, annual review *167*

dementia *181–187*
dementia assessment *182, 185*
dementia diagnosis *182–185*
dementia, types of *184*
dengue fever *71*
depression *176, 177*
diabetes *52, 107–130, 162, 163*
diabetes complications *122, 123, 124*

diabetes, diagnosis *108, 110, 111*
diabetes management *113–129*
diabetes prevention *112*
diabetes risk factors *113*
diabetic ketoacidosis (DKA) *126*
diabetic nephropathy *124*
diabetic neuropathy *124*
diabetic retinopathy *123*
diphtheria *60*
disease prevention *2*
dyspnoea scale *140*

ear candles *80*
ear care *77–82*
ear self-care *78, 79*
ear syringing *77, 81*
ear syringing, complications *81*
ear wax removal *77, 78, 79*
end of life care *177, 187*
erectile dysfunction (ED) *52*
exercise referral *121*

family planning service *37*
female genital mutilation (FGM) *39*
FEV1/FVC ratio *138*
fractional exhaled nitric oxide (FeNO) *139*
'free-rider' problem *58*

General Practice Workforce Development Plan *6*
glycaemic control *114, 163*
GPN, changing role of *1–7*
GPN role, 1960s-1980s *2*
GPN role, 2000-2010 *3*
GPN role, 2010 onwards *4*

Haemophilus influenzae type b (Hib) 61
Health Belief Model 23
health inequalities 20
health literacy 24
health promotion 2, 22
health screening 17–24
healthcare assistants (HCAs) 3
heart failure 165, 166, 167
Hepatitis B 61
herd immunity 56, 57
home blood glucose monitoring (HBGM) 118
hormones, menstrual 36
House of Care 101, 102
HPV triage 31
human papilloma virus (HPV) 29
hypercholesterolaemia 161
hyperosmolar hyperglycaemic state (HHS) 128
hypertension 160, 161
hypoglycaemia 127

immunisation 55–66, 70
immunisations, administration of 65
immunisation schedules 63, 64, 65
immunity 59
infection 93
inhaled steroids (IHSs) 142, 143
inhaler devices 145, 146
insulin therapy 125

leukotriene-receptor antagonists 144
lifestyle change 114
long-term conditions 97–103
long-term medical conditions and women 39

Making Every Contact Count 23

maintenance and reliever therapy (MART) 144
malaria 71
measles 62
medication reviews 199
memory service 185
Meningitis C 61
men's health 45–53
menstrual cycle 35, 36
mental illness 103, 189–194
mental illness, effects of 190
mental illness in children and adolescents 191
mental illness, incidence of 190
mental illness, prevention of 192
mental illness, types of 191, 192
metformin 113
MMR vaccination 56
mosquito bites, avoiding 71, 72
mucolytics 145
multimorbidity 174
mumps 62
myocardial infarction (MI) 163

Neighbour's model 14
NMC Code 197, 198

obesity 159
oral anticoagulation therapy (OAC) 164
overweight 159
ovulation 36

pain management 175
pain relief ladder 176
palliative care 177, 187
patient education 114
patient group direction 200
patient satisfaction 15
patient specific direction 201
peak expiratory flow variability 139

Pendleton's model 14
personalised care planning 100
pertussis 61
phosphodiesterase type-4 inhibitors 145
Pneumococcal infection 62
polio 61
Prehn's sign 50
prostate 46
prostate cancer 46–48
prostate cancer risk stratification 47
prostate-specific antigen (PSA) 46
public health 17–24
public health agencies 18
Public Health Agency Northern Ireland 20
public health challenges 17
public health domains 18
Public Health England 19
Public Health Wales 21

quality of life 98
Queen's Nursing Institute 5

reflection 15
respiratory conditions 133–148
respiratory disease management 140
respiratory disease medications 141
risk assessment for travel 70, 71
rotavirus 62
rubella 62

Scotland, health in 22
screening criteria 27
scrotal swelling 49
sedentary lifestyle 159
self-care in long-term conditions 98, 99

self-management *99*
skin, function of *85*
skin, layers of *87*
smear test, taking *31*
smoking *162, 190*
Social Cognitive Theory *23*
Social Ecological Models *23*
spirometry *137, 138*
Stages of Change Model *23*
statins *161*
suicide *190*

testes, self-examination of *51*
testicular cancer *49–52*
testicular torsion *49*
tetanus *61*
transillumination *50*
Transtheoretical Model *23*
travel health *69–75*
type 2 diabetes diagnosis *110*

vaccination, contraindications *65*
vaccination controversies *56*
vaccination planner *63*
vaccination programme, aim of *58*
vaccination side effects *66*
vaccinations, travel-related *69, 70*

Wakefield Study *56*

weight loss measures *115*
whooping cough *61*
women's health *35–42*
women's health, sociocultural factors in *41*
wound assessment *88, 89, 90*
wound care *85–94*
wound dressing *91, 92*
wound healing *86, 87, 88*
wound infection *93*
wounds, types of *86*

xanthines *144*

yellow fever *71*

zika virus *71*